# the DMSO handbook

# the DMSO handbook

A Complete Guide to the History and use of DMSO

Halstead &
Youngberg

Golden Quill Publishers, Inc.

FIRST EDITION, JUNE 1981



**GOLDEN QUILL PUBLISHERS, INC.**
**P.O. BOX 1278**
**COLTON, CA 92324**
**(714) 783-0119**

LIBRARY OF CONGRESS CATALOG CARD NUMBER: 81-82387

INTERNATIONAL STANDARD BOOK NUMBER
0-933904-07-X PAPERBACK
0-933904-08-8 HARDBACK

MEMBER
COSMEP
COMMITTEE OF SMALL MAGAZINE EDITORS AND PUBLISHERS
BOX 703 SAN FRANCISCO, CA 9410

# Dedication

This handbook is dedicated to the men and women of medicine and science who feel it is their duty and their right to seek the truth, despite the political, social, and professional pressures they might encounter. It is their steadfast dedication to these ends that we humbly salute.

# Acknowledgements

This book is the literary crystallization of the thoughts, studies, and work of many people known and unknown to the authors. Therefore it is impossible to fully acknowledge everyone who has contributed to the study of DMSO which made this book possible. We owe a great deal to the many diligent investigators of DMSO who were undaunted in their efforts to seek the truth even in the face of great adversity and scorn.

We are indebted to the work of Dr. Stanley Jacob and Robert Herschler who initiated the original studies on DMSO in the treatment of disease and also the AG Schering Corporation of Europe for their academic contributions. We would also like to recognize the New York Academy of Sciences who sponsored two international symposia on DMSO despite overwhelming political and social pressures. Without their insight and vision, DMSO may have never seen the light of day.

We would like to thank Loretta L. Hood for her excellent advice and technical help in preparing this manuscript.

We are also grateful to Jennine M. Vinci, who typed and retyped the manuscript through its many drafts, and to Kay Martinez (Kay Martinez Typesetting Service) who typeset and prepared the finished product for publication.

# Contents

# Preface

This *DMSO Handbook* was prepared in reply to the request of many of our medical colleagues and patients who were forever asking, "What is this DMSO stuff all about?" This book was not intended to be an exhaustive, technical monograph, but rather a practical workbook for both the practitioner and consumer. The sections on chemistry, pharmacology, and toxicology go into greater technical depth in order to provide the interested reader with some insight as to scientific reasons for the mechanisms of action of this phenomenal compound.

Our present knowledge as to all of the mechanisms of action of DMSO is still unknown. However, this same statement can be made for numerous other highly effective therapeutic agents. Although pharmacodynamic principles are always desirable and important, it is not imperative that they be fully delineated before the compound is used clinically.

We have used DMSO over the past several years at the Halstead Preventive Medical Clinic in Loma Linda, California, in the treatment of hundreds of patients for a wide range of ailments. At times, we have been disappointed because we failed to achieve all the therapeutic results desired; but more times than not we have been pleasantly surprised to find DMSO has brought relief of pain and objective clinical improvements when all other modalities have failed. We have never observed any negative effects related to its safety and toxicity.

The history of the development of DMSO reads like a novel and the FDA has been overly cooperative in providing all of the intrigue one might expect in a good novel. A critical review of the FDA's dealing with DMSO clearly reveals an inappropriate use of its regulatory powers and a duplicity in the application of drug standards, both as to efficacy and toxicity. One has merely to refer to the *Physician's Desk Reference* (PDR) and examine most of the drugs that have been approved by the FDA in order to see the disparity and unequal application of drug standards and laws. The FDA appears to follow one set of standards for drugs they wish to approve and an entirely different set for those they wish to keep off the market.

DMSO has been aptly termed "the persecuted drug." The incongruity of standards governing new drug approval in the United States is one of the greatest threats to the health and welfare of its citizenry. The "new-drug-approval" game can hardly be ascribed to the mere bungling of an inept bureaucratic federal agency. Unfortunately it involves a great deal of malice aforethought by a regulatory body that needs to be brought in line with the best health interests of the nation. The past performance of the FDA was first a regulatory decision, then a political stance, and then the assemblage of technical data to back a position on a drug that has become a political and legal "hot potato." This type of performance does not constitute good science. The mishandling of DMSO has cost this nation an untold amount of needless pain and misery, unwarranted medical expenses to the patient-consumer, and an untold loss in lives due to the failure of the medical establishment to take advantage of a remarkable therapeutic agent.

Once upon a time there was a revolutionary Surgeon General by the name of Benjamin Rush. He was said to be very prominent and influential, but highly controversial. He was not greatly admired by some of his medical peers. Nevertheless, he, among others, appended his signature to a document. One of the statements in this historical document reads as follows: "We hold these truths to be self-evident, that all men are created equal, that they are endowed by their Creator with certain inalienable Rights, that among these are Life, Liberty, and the pursuit of Happiness . . . That when any form of Government becomes destructive of these ends, it is the right of the people to alter or to abolish it, and to institute new Government . . ."

It is our belief that this arm of government has become "destructive of these ends." The history of DMSO is a case history of medical depotism by a governmental agency. It is our sincerest desire in writing this book to not only shed some light on the subject of DMSO, but in so doing perhaps take a step in "altering" an agency of our government which has veered from the objectives it was established to pursue in the service of the people.

Bruce W. Halstead, M.D.
Sylvia A. Youngberg, R.N.

February, 1981

# A Word About DMSO

Ever since 37 million Americans recently viewed an explosive segment on the popular television series *60 Minutes* on DMSO, the "medical wonder of our age," the flurry of excitement has never abated. Never has any substance with such "miraculous" therapeutic capabilities met with such an overwhelming barrage of enthusiasm on the one hand and controversy and skepticism on the other. Practically overnight it has become one of the hottest blackmarket drugs to have ever swept the country. It is being made available in such unlikely places as flea markets, candy stores, hobby shops, and dry cleaners. A person unfamiliar with the undercurrents surrounding DMSO might question why a drug of this magnitude would not be available at the corner drugstore.

The major reason stems from the fact that the governmental regulatory agency, the Food and Drug Administration, has persisted in following a very close-minded course through the past 15 years despite thousands of scientific articles and several international symposia on DMSO and its efficacy and safety.

This enduringly negative and passive stance assumed by the FDA, coupled with the universal need for education and exposure to the unbiased information on DMSO, has created a need for factual presentation about the drug.

Dimethyl sulfoxide, more popularly known as DMSO, first discovered in Russia in 1866, is undoubtedly one of the most remarkable compounds to be discovered during the past century. The medical applications of DMSO have been the subject of four international conferences. The first was held in West Berlin in 1965 under the aegis of the German pharmaceutical company Schering AG. Then in 1966, the New York Academy of Sciences sponsored a conference. The third conference was held in Vienna under the auspices of Schering AG and the University of Vienna Medical School. The fourth conference was sponsored by the New York Academy of Sciences in 1975.

In 1973, the United States National Academy of Sciences and the Division of Medical Sciences of the National Research Council under contract with the Food and Drug Administration reviewed approximately 1,200 foreign and domestic research papers and more than 193 volumes of special reports submitted to the FDA by manufacturers and independent investigators dealing with various laboratory and clinical aspects of DMSO therapy in humans and laboratory animals.

Despite the enormous flurry of scientific activity concerning the chemistry, pharmacology, toxicology, and clinical efficacy of DMSO, it continues to be the most controversial drug today, exclusive of laetrile. More than 100 years have lapsed since the discovery of DMSO. It is estimated that since the rediscovery and the initiation of the application of DMSO beginning about 1960 with the work of Stanley W. Jacob, M.D. and Robert J. Herschler, more than six million individuals have used DMSO as a therapeutic agent without any significant, verified evidence of toxicity. In addition, millions of Americans have been purchasing DMSO from a disorganized array of non-medical retailers. Therefore, it is anyone's guess as to how many millions of persons have used DMSO in the last few decades. Although this is poor science, it is significant that no toxicity reports have come out of this unsupervised DMSO medication movement.

Dimethyl sulfoxide is a wood pulp derivative. Its precursor can be obtained from milk, tomatoes, cooked corn, asparagus, clams, tea, coffee, and other substances. It can be made from many organic bases. The process by which DMSO is made commercially involves the reaction of a black lignin-bearing liquor from the digestion in the kraft pulp process with molten sulfur. This produces dimethyl sulfide which is then oxidized with nitrogen tetroxide to yield dimethyl sulfoxide.

DMSO is rapidly absorbed and distributed in living tissues, loses its oxygen, and is excreted in part as dimethyl sulfide, which provides the garlic-like odor to the breath. Studies with radioactive sulfur in DMSO show that sulfur from the compound may remain in the body for several days.

Extensive toxicity studies have been conducted using single and repeated dosages of DMSO in humans and on a variety of laboratory animals. Single intravenous doses as high as one gram per kilogram of body weight in dogs have failed to show any significant untoward effects (Smith, Hadidian, and Mason, 1968). Although ocular damage has been reported in some laboratory animals due to the prolonged use of DMSO, no eye damage has been reported in humans.

DMSO possesses both radioprotective and cryoprotective properties. The precise mechanisms involved are not completely known.

DMSO has been used with varying degrees of success in a great variety of medical ailments, including burns, musculoskeletal traumatic injuries, bursitis, arthritis, cancer, scleroderma, urinary tract disorders, osteomyelitis, cerebral edema, neurological disorders, multiple sclerosis, cardiovascular diseases, respiratory disorders, herpes, mental retardation, and a variety of infectious processes, etc. The therapeutic spectrum has curiously been a major drawback, seriously affecting the credibility of clinicians working with the compound. However, DMSO is not a panacea. A study of the chemistry and pharmacology of DMSO begins to shed some light on the scientific basis of its mechanism of action and why this drug is able to possess such a broad therapeutic spectrum. Physicians who have had extensive clinical experience with DMSO over the past 10 to 15 years not only vehemently extol its therapeutic efficacy in the treatment of various ailments, but also testify to its phenomenal toxicological safety.

Perhaps the late Chauncey D. Leake, the famous pharmacologist, (1966) summed up the situation quite succinctly when he stated at the symposium on DMSO held by the New York Academy of Sciences in 1966, " . . . rarely has a new drug come so quickly to the judgment of the members of the health professions with so much verifiable data from so many parts of the world, both experimentally and clinically, as to safety and efficacy." Leake's commentary appears to have fallen on deaf ears and blind observers as far as the FDA is concerned because now, 15 years later, the medical bureaucracy is still as incapable of making a decision on the DMSO matter as they were before they undertook their first evaluation in the early 1960's. The FDA appears to be suffering from a rare form of "scientific myopia" that not even copious quantities of DMSO can cure.

In the text that follows, no attempt has been made to provide an exhaustive review of the vast assemblage of scientific literature on DMSO, but a sincere attempt has been made to provide a thorough review of the major highlights concerning the chemistry, pharmacology, and clinical applications of this most remarkable of all therapeutic agents. Hopefully this data will provide a useful scientific insight to professionals and laymen alike.

# 1

# A Historical Perspective

Dimethyl sulfoxide, more commonly known as DMSO, was first synthesized in 1866 in the eastern Russian city of Kasan, Tatar Republic, on the Volga River. The discoverer was a chemist named Alexander M. Saytzeff. He found this substance, a wood pulp derivative, to be colorless and clear, much like water. It was bitter tasting and left a garlicky, oyster-like aftertaste and odor. When the slightly viscuous solution was applied to the skin, it left it warm and slightly dry. Most remarkable, however, was its ability to dissolve other substances that were combined with it.

**Initial discovery**

Saytzeff wrote an article in March, 1866, describing the process whereby "dimethylschwefeloxyd" (DMSO) is synthesized by oxidation of dimethyl sulfide. This article appeared in a journal published in Germany in 1867 and was entitled *"ueber die Einwirkung von Salpersaure auf Schwefelmethyl und Schwefelathyl"* (Saytzeff, 1867).

**First article published**

For roughly eight decades, scientists failed to explore Saytzeff's rudimentary findings. It was shortly after the

Second World War that industrial researchers around the world began investigating the solvent capabilities of DMSO. Initially, the knowledge obtained was concerned with the physical properties of DMSO. About this time a worldwide research endeavor was undertaken to utilize forest-derived waste chemicals. The research turned to a more practical nature in an effort to produce a superior synthetic fiber. Improved solvents for dyes, resins, paints, and agriculture chemicals were needed. DMSO began to receive closer scrutiny. By 1948, its physiochemical properties began to emerge (Rosenbaum and Jacob, 1964).

**Solvent capabilities identified**

Commercial development of DMSO was initially undertaken about 1953. Production in the United States was initiated by the Stephan Chemical Company of Chicago and Crown Zellerbach Corporation, a large paper manufacturing company. These companies promoted DMSO as a superior solvent. In 1959, a massive explosion occurred at the Stephan Chemical plant which ended further research and commercial development of DMSO by their company. Crown Zellerbach Corporation then became the only U.S. producer of DMSO. During this same year, Crown began construction of a new plant in Bongalusa, Louisiana, in order to expand their production capabilities of DMSO and related products (Block, 1964).

**Commercial development undertaken**

**Crown Zellerbach becomes only U.S. producer**

The biological properties of DMSO began to emerge in 1959 when Lovelock and Bishop reported on their successful substitution of DMSO for ethylene glycon, an anti-freeze additive. This property of DMSO was later used to protect animal and human living cells from damage by freezing (Lovelock and Bishop, 1959).

**Biological properties discovered**

Robert J. Herschler was the Supervisor of Applications Research in the Chemical Products Division at the Crown Zellerbach plant in Camas, Washington. By 1960, he had worked for Crown approximately twenty years. He had been conducting research on interesting chemicals, one of which was DMSO. He felt that some of these substances might be of value in other areas of science, especially medicine. Once, when basic dyes containing DMSO had been accidentally spilled in the laboratory, he noted that the color appeared to penetrate very deeply into the worker's skin. Furthermore, he noted that when a pesticide solution of DDT and DMSO was spilled, those contaminated became sick. Herschler went on to discover that DMSO combined with antifungal and antibiotic agents penetrated the surface of plants resulting in better growth without blight infestation or fungus development. He concluded that DMSO might be useful in the treatment of plant disease.

**Herschler's initial experiments**

**Jacob's landmark discoveries**

Stanley W. Jacob, M.D., was an Assistant Professor of Surgery at the University of Oregon Medical School in Portland, Oregon, where he had been performing experimental organ transplants on dogs. He was looking for a means to preserve organs for transplant, so that when they were needed, they could be immediately implanted. He had stored living organs under high pressures in a cold environment and had also used various anti-freezing agents. However, nothing seemed to prevent the formation of the ice crystals that altered delicate tissue in the organs. Jacob later read a British report on the success of using DMSO as a preservative for bone marrow and for blood. This prompted him to begin research on the physical and chemical properties of DMSO.

**Medical research begins**

Late in 1961, Herschler and Jacob met at the University of Oregon Medical School and began discussing DMSO and some of the exciting possibilities of the substance. The fire of enthusiasm regarding DMSO was then kindled; medical research on DMSO had begun (McGrady, 1973).

**Clinical trials prove successful**

These two scientists began experimenting with the use of DMSO as a vehicle to promote the penetration of antibiotics into third-degree burn wounds in rats, to speed healing, and reduce infection. The results were successful; animal survival was prolonged and it appeared to enhance healing as well. Then DMSO was given to a patient following a chemical burn and it not only promoted rapid healing, but also relieved pain. It was also noted by the laboratory personnel that topical application of DMSO relieved the pain of bruises, muscle strain, and ecchymoses. It also reduced swelling and seemed to hasten recovery (NAS, 1973).

**Publishing attempts fail**

By the summer of 1963, Jacob and Herschler had compiled a summary of the basic pharmacological properties of DMSO. This summary was then submitted to *Nature*, *Surgery*, and *Science* for publication. All three publications turned their paper down insisting that their claims were preposterous. In October, 1963, Jacob presented his findings on DMSO before the Surgical Biology Club at the University of Oregon. They too were amused at what they considered to be his "rare brand of humor." They refused to allow him to present his report to the Society of University Surgeons.

The prospects for medical recognition of DMSO appeared bleak. Regretfully, this situation is not new to medicine or to science. Doubt, scorn, and even persecution were not uncommon to men such as Galileo, Pasteur, Semmelweis, and Galen, as well as many other reknown medical researchers. Stumbling blocks of this nature have delayed major scientific advancement since time immemorial and continue to plague mankind to this day.

**Patent sought**

On December 9, 1963, partnership papers for the patent on the medical use of DMSO were applied for by the Oregon Board of Higher Education (Jacob's assignor) and by Crown Zellerbach Corporation (Herschler's assignor). The application was filed at the Oregon State Capitol in Salem. Simultaneously, the DMSO "claims" and properties became open to the public and the press. Local papers in Portland carried the story on page one the following day and within a week the story had traversed the nation. *The New York Times* gave it page one recognition on December 18. Crown Zellerbach stock jumped as *Newsweek*, *U.S. News and World Report*, *Life*, and *Saturday Evening Post* distributed accounts which touted prospects for the future of DMSO.

**DMSO receives worldwide publicity**

By 1964, DMSO was beginning to attain respectability at last. Medical and scientific periodicals began publishing papers on DMSO. Clinical trials were being conducted in many new and challenging areas. Animal trials were confirming the biological safety of DMSO. In March, 1964, the FDA met with representatives of Crown Zellerbach and the University of Oregon and seemed anxious to assist in the continued testing of DMSO. They advised, after one month's toxicity data was completed at Oregon State Hospital, that human clinical trials could begin in earnest.

**FDA approves human experimentation**

Initially, the pharmaceutical companies were skeptical about DMSO, then curious, then, finally, interested. However, there were mixed feelings; DMSO was an inexpensive product and it could possibly substitute for a very large number of pharmaceuticals that had cost their industry vast sums of money to develop. Nevertheless, drug house enthusiasm about DMSO slowly began to intensify. Interested firms included Geigy, Squibb, Syntex, Merck, and the American Shering Corporation. As the FDA's demands on DMSO testing standards became more stringent, the cost of laboratory equipment and clinical testing began skyrocketing. Initially, the estimated cost was $10 million, then it rose to $15 million and beyond. It very well could be one of the drug industry's most invested-in and most investigated drugs.

**Drug companies become interested**

The first international symposium on the DMSO drug concept was held in West Berlin, Germany, on July 2, 1965. It was sponsored by Schering AG, a German drug house. There were approximately 150 participants representing various European nations. The Germans, even though they had begun their studies later than those initiated in the U.S., made very impressive presentations in the area of scientific data.

**First international symposium staged**

On September 8, 1965, Merck, Sharp, and Dohme Laboratories sent an advisory memorandum to all investigators of DMSO enumerating the medicinal prospects of the drug since the release of DMSO as a prescription drug appeared imminent. Merck's initial clinical studies included over 4,000 patients who had received DMSO over periods of up to 18 months.

Then, on September 9, 1965, the *Wall Street Journal* reported that a lady in Ireland had died from an allergic reaction to DMSO. This was the first indication that DMSO might produce allergic reactions or dangerous side effects.

**Dangerous side effects feared**

In the press release significant facts regarding this fatality were omitted. This 44-year-old woman had taken an estimated total of only 30ml of DMSO over a 3-day period for a sprained wrist and knee. She had been taking penicillin, a drug responsible for many deaths due to allergies each year, as well as an unnamed drug prescribed to combat depression. Her symptoms were tongue swelling and choking. After her death, no autopsy was performed. One would question why the emphasis was placed solely on DMSO as the cause of death, considering the medical facts.

**FDA halts testing**

Then, on November 11, 1965, clinical testing of DMSO in the United States was brought to an abrupt halt by the FDA. Laboratory testing of DMSO had caused refractory lens changes to occur in three species of animals not closely related to humans. These unfavorable effects were reversed when DMSO was terminated. Importantly, no eye changes had ever been noted in humans.

**Refractory lens changes observed**

Two weeks after the FDA blocked further testing of DMSO, almost all FDA inspectors were called back to Washington, the largest recall of inspectors in history. At the briefing, the inspectors were informed that there was serious question as to whether the FDA had been correct in halting DMSO testing because of animal toxicity. The plan was now to go out into the field and find "pigeons" so they could prove the physicians investigating DMSO to be dishonest. They must also find disgruntled patients that had experienced adverse side effects after DMSO treatment who would testify before Congressional committees. The

**FDA plan to block DMSO research**

physicians investigating the drug would be tried in the press. Within the FDA organization there was considerable competition for promotions. The agents had not forgotten that Dr. Kelsey had received recognition and a medal for stopping thalidomide, a drug that caused deformity in unborn children.

In late November, 1965, FDA agents appeared at Jacob and Rosenbaum's offices and began copying patient records—they both were doing clinical research with DMSO in Portland at the time. However, by December Jacob noted they were also copying personal correspondence as well. Jacob requested that their personal correspondence photocopies be destroyed. He was told that since government equipment had been used by government agents on government time, they could not destroy government property.

**Jacob and Rosenbaum investigated by FDA**

The University of Oregon Medical School filed a protest against the actions of the FDA agents. Fundamental rights of a citizen as guaranteed by the Constitution had been violated, not to mention breaches of the sacred physician-patient relationship. The agents were acting far beyond the scope of authority delegated to them.

**Protest against FDA filed**

The FDA, realizing it needed to expand its controls, asked Congress for police powers over scientists and physicians. The Commissioner presented his case against DMSO on March 9, 1966, at a hearing before the House of Representatives Fountain Subcommittee on Drug Safety.

Dr. Goddard, the newly appointed FDA Commissioner who prior to this position had been in private practice as a physician for a total of only sixteen months, was about to wield unprecendented, almost dictatorial power over the medical profession. He asked Congress to give the FDA the authority to become a surveillant over the clinical investigators. He told the Committee, "We are investigating possible criminal violations" in the clinical research of DMSO. Furthermore, there had been "at least one death"—the lady in Ireland. These statements made headlines throughout the

**FDA seeks stricter controls**

United States. Notably absent from the Congressional hearing was any testimony as to whether DMSO actually was detrimental or beneficial.

**Congress grants FDA new powers**

The Congressional Subcommittee granted four amendments to the Narcotic and Drug Abuse Act adopted in February, 1960. Notably, the FDA agents were given authority to seize, with or without libels of information, execute and serve search warrants, serve arrests, even make arrests without warrants in certain cases, and carry firearms.

These generous police power endowments given to the FDA were purported to be measures to promote drug safety to a degree unsurpassed anywhere in the world. No thought was given to the stifling of the future development of drugs as well as the halting of scientific progress. It appeared that the FDA had been given formidable policing powers similar to that of the Gestapo.

In 1966, the New York Academy made plans for a symposium on DMSO despite efforts made by the FDA and the drug industry to prevent it. A symposium which exposed the true facts on DMSO could prove very embarrassing to the FDA. A great credit must go to those arranging the symposium for not allowing political and economical considerations to compromise the search for scientific truth.

**New York Academy symposium held**

The New York Academy had over 27,000 members throughout the United States and in many foreign countries. It sponsored meetings for a vast array of scientific disciplines. In preparation for the symposium, letters were sent around the world seeking abstracts on DMSO studies for presentation. In an effort to maintain balance, a specific attempt was made to find negative papers. However, it was virtually impossible to find unfavorable reports from knowledgeable scientists.

The New York Academy of Sciences held their symposium on DMSO on March 14, 15, and 16, 1966, at the large hall of New York's Waldorf Astorial Hotel. One of the most respected and powerful figures in medical education, Dr. Chauncey Leake, of the University of California Medical Center, chaired the symposium. Now deceased, Dr. Chauncey Leake has been called the Dean of American pharmacologists. Eighty-two scheduled papers were presented. Many additional extemporaneous speeches were made as well. The main emphasis of the symposium dealt with the toxicology and pharmacology of DMSO. Papers were also presented on the ability of DMSO to protect living cells from lethal damage by cold and radiation. The clinical spectrum of the diseases covered was far greater than that which had ever been considered in the past in respect to a single drug.

**Symposium papers published**

The papers presented at the session were published in a 671 page volume, *Annals of the New York Academy of Sciences,* Vol. 141, Art. 1. *Biological Actions of Dimethyl Sulfoxide*, March 15, 1967.

**Third international symposium—Austria**

On November 8 and 9, 1966, the third international symposium was held at the Palais Pallavicini in Vienna, Austria. It was financed by Shering AG, a major German pharmaceutical company, and sponsored by the University of Vienna Medical School. One hundred fifty scientists from twelve countries attended. Papers were submitted on the action of DMSO as related to a large variety of diseases. As in the case of the previous New York and Berlin symposia, scientists reported that DMSO failed to cause eye damage in humans or in any primate animal species. Members of the health profession throughout the world were becoming increasingly wary of judgments made by the U.S. Food and Drug Administration.

**Discussions and reports published**

The discussions and reports at the Vienna conference were published and distributed by Shering AG of Germany. The book, entitled *Dimethyl-sulfoxide–DMSO, Internationales Symposium,* contained fine color photographs, particularly of the reversible eye changes in certain species of animals (Laudahn and Gertich, 1966).

**FDA approves limited testing**

In December, 1966, the FDA began to allow a limited resumption of clinical testing in the United States on DMSO. However the harrassment by the agency continued. Agents entered Crown Zellerbach's warehouses and smashed bottles of DMSO. One of the officers at the plant, a German refugee, was said to have remarked that the FDA operations were reminiscent of Gestapo tactics. An officer at Pfizer, a major drug house, was grilled by FDA agents repeatedly. They questioned whether there had been collusion between scientists and drug houses to hide the toxicity of DMSO or make unwarranted therapeutic claims.

**Vacaville experiments**

In October, 1967, the FDA granted E. R. Squibb and Sons permission for controlled testing of DMSO on humans. Dr. Richard Brobyn, a young physician at Bainbridge Medical Center in Washington, conducted the study. The group selected to be studied consisted of sixty-seven healthy male prisoners at the California Medical Facility in Vacaville. Before DMSO was administered, very extensive examinations were performed on each man. These included bone marrow punctures, spinal taps, eye, heart, and brain studies, as well as numerous blood, urine and other body fluid tests. An initial two-week course of DMSO was begun. The tests were repeated and then a three-month study was conducted that comprised one of the largest and most competent toxicological studies ever undertaken. Each man received 1gm/kg of DMSO, three to thirty times the normal therapeutic dose, administered in an 80 percent gel concentration and applied daily. They were tested and inspected on a regular basis, as were a separate group of men in a control group. The study concluded that no prisoner-volunteer had shown evidence of any serious toxic effects from DMSO. There was no evidence of eye damage. The side effects reported were identical to those seen by many physicians previously: breath and skin odor, skin irritation, and occasional headaches. DMSO was found to be amazingly gentle, even at many times the ordinary dose (Brobyn, 1975).

The cost of this study, $90,000, was split between

Squibb and the FDA. It was a classic in toxicology. However, while the experiment gave DMSO a remarkably clean bill of health in relation to its safety, no significant changes in the status of DMSO resulted.

Finally, in September, 1968, the FDA issued new regulations which eliminated many of the restrictions regarding the use of DMSO in clinical trials. These regulations allowed it to be used for investigational purposes with patients suffering from musculoskeletal disorders and not to exceed 14 days per treatment.

**FDA relaxes restrictions**

In 1970, the FDA approved the use of DMSO in the treatment of horses by veterinarians. Use was limited to not more than 100ml applied topically daily for a maximum of thirty days and was specifically restricted to use with non-breeding horses.

**Veterinary use approved**

On December 22, 1970, the United States Patent Office issued Patent No. 3,549,770 for "Therapeutic Administration of Effective Amounts of Dimethyl Sulfoxide to Human and Animal Subjects." The patent covered thirty-seven claims and is said to represent the broadest approval given to a medicinal agent by the United States Patent Office (Herschler and Jacob, 1970).

**Patent issued**

Ironically, the Patent Office was honoring claims made for DMSO by Herschler and Jacob, albeit seven years after filing, while the FDA was still banning the use of the substance.

Under contract with the FDA, the National Academy of Sciences—National Research Council formed an *ad hoc* Committee on Dimethyl Sulfoxide in 1972. The purpose of the study was to review all available scientific data as to the clinical effectiveness and toxicity of DMSO, and determine if the FDA restrictions on the drug were appropriate.

**NAS-NRC study began**

In August of 1973, the NAS-NRC study was completed.

**Positive study results obtained**

They released a 119-page summary of their investigation referring specifically to 230 reports and listing a bibliography of about 300. They concluded by stating that the FDA had been overly restrictive in regard to DMSO and that the toxicological data did not warrant withholding the drug. However, they stated that more clinical trials should be undertaken to determine its therapeutic value and toxicity before being generally released as a prescriptive drug (NAS, 1973).

**Book on DMSO published**

In 1973, Doubleday released a book written by Pat McGrady, Sr., entitled *The Persecuted Drug: The Story of DMSO*, in which the saga of DMSO and the FDA was vividly and entertainingly chronicled (McGrady, 1973). This book explained with objective thoroughness not only the efficacy of DMSO, but also detailed the efforts of the Food and Drug Administration to justify its rulings. It would appear that the agency would rather prevent the use of a highly efficacious drug than expose themselves to possible criticism for their prior actions.

**Fourth international symposium—New York**

The fourth international symposium on DMSO was held in New York on January 9, 10, and 11, 1974, again under the sponsorship of the erudite New York Academy of Sciences. Dr. Chauncey Leake, in his opening remarks at the conference, commented that the FDA operates under an act "which seems to imply that no drug is to be used by a physician unless it is demonstrated to be absolutely safe and absolutely effective." "There is no such drug," he added, "not even tap water or table salt are absolutely safe and effective" (Leake, 1975).

Eighty-two papers were presented at the symposium representing research being conducted around the world. Again, the researchers were virtually unanimous in their findings: DMSO was effective in a host of diseases and there was only negligible toxicity.

**Symposium papers published**

The papers presented at the symposium were published in January, 1975, in the *Annals of the New York Academy of*

*Sciences*, Vol. 243, *Biological Actions of Dimethyl Sulfoxide.*

In 1978, after a struggle of more than a decade, the FDA finally approved the prescriptive use of DMSO for the treatment of interstitial cystitis, a rare bladder disease. Medical grade DMSO became available from Research Industries in Utah, a division of Merck, under the name of Rimso-50. This sterile, pyrogen-free, 50 percent strength solution of DMSO is still available for use.

**Prescriptive use of DMSO approved**

In 1980, the FDA rejected the request of the Arthritis Advisory Committee to make DMSO available for scleroderma. In a recent *FDA Drug Bulletin* on DMSO they stated, "Studies to determine the effectiveness of DMSO are under way for other conditions, including muscle sprains and strains, several urologic conditions, acute spinal cord injury, and stroke" (FDA, 1980).

**Use for scleroderma rejected**

In March, 1980, the television program *60 Minutes* reported on DMSO and its controversial history before a viewing audience of approximately 37 million people. The DMSO segment received possibly the largest viewer response in the program's 12-year history (Bergreen, 1980).

***60 Minutes***

Again in 1980, DMSO was brought to the attention of Congress. The House Select Committee on Aging, headed by Committee Chairman Claude Pepper (D-Fla.), re-evaluated DMSO. While Dr. Crout stated he would be willing to co-operate with the Committee, he did state that "There is no evidence that DMSO has altered the course of any disease."

**Congress re-evaluates DMSO**

The reasons why the FDA has been overly restrictive on DMSO are not clear. Perhaps it could be too embarrassing for the agency to retract their previously staunch position. There are many other instances in which their patience has been inappropriately monumental. Even though science in these instances has presented them with sufficient evidence as to the hazards of certain dangerous drugs and foods, they have postponed taking action for years, as illustrated by these

**FDA's activities questioned**

few examples:

- the carcinogenic effect of sodium cyclamate and sacchrin;
- the brain lesions in animals injected with monosodium glutamate;
- the unrestricted use of methotrexate after at least twenty-five deaths were attributed to its toxicity;
- delaying action on diethylstilbesterol (DES) for eight months after reports indicating pregnant women treated with it bore girl babies with a tendency to develop a rare vaginal cancer. And despite the urging of physicians and public, DES was allowed to be given to cattle and poultry to fatten them for many years after DES was banned for human use.

**Abuse of regulatory powers**

For years the agency has been criticized bitterly by those familiar with its operations. Its regulatory power has not been administered in a flexible or scientific manner. Because of this, applications for the Investigation of New Drugs, IND's, submitted to the agency have steadily and drastically declined in recent years, thus stifling scientific progress. The fallacy that the FDA is the protector of the people continues to be believed by the masses, although evidence is growing that the agency is not properly informing or protecting consumers. The FDA has evolved from a position of obscurity into the world's largest regulator of consumer goods. Unfortunately, in so doing, it has gained a reputation as the United States government's most demoralized, fractionalized, and criticized agency. Its far-reaching powers have burgeoned as has its budget of well over $312 million a year.

**Effects of ban**

In evaluating the management of DMSO, it seems absurd that there was no consumers' advocate, no intermediate arm of government, no press, no lobby, nor voluntary health agency to protest. The pharmaceutical industry accepted the ban with quiet resignation; they were rid of a relatively cheap, but superior product which would have competed with their expensive wares. Unfortunately, the only cries of protest were from distraught patients. Though amateurish and sparse in numbers, angry patients attempted to be heard so they could continue the DMSO therapy so essential to their health and well-being. It is impossible to determine the number of patients who died unnecessarily, became paralyzed or bedridden when DMSO became so abruptly unavailable. It is encouraging to note, however, that for many years DMSO has been available as a prescriptive drug (in some areas for over twelve years) in Switzerland, West Germany, the Soviet Union, Austria, Great Britian, Ireland, China, Mexico, Canada, and in several South American countries.

**Countries where DMSO is available**

It would be preposterous to maintain that no FDA is needed in our country today. The FDA has definately made a positive contribution in the management of the food and pharmaceutical industry, contributing to the health and welfare of the citizens of the United States. They have exerted much needed protective controls over such substances as food dyes, DDT, a host of toxins, as well as other dangerous food additives, drugs, and chemical agents. Unfortunately, they have been inconsistent in their regulatory management, as exemplified by their approval of numerous drugs which bear a long list of devastating side effects and contraindications. Comparatively, DMSO has a wide margin of safety, yet has met with continual repression by this Agency. One can only hope that as the remarkable therapeutic attributes of DMSO become more widely recognized, the Food and Drug Administration will enthusiastically lend its endorsement.

**Agency reforms needed**

# 2

# A Chemical Overview

Dimethyl sulfoxide (DMSO) is one of the most versatile substances among organic sulfur compounds and in organic chemistry in general. The chemistry of DMSO is now well established and a vast volume of scientific literature is available on the subject. However, since much of this chemical data is more directly related to the industrial uses of DMSO, this presentation will deal primarily with those aspects that have a bearing on its mechanism of action as a therapeutic agent.

**DMSO as a therapeutic agent**

DMSO is commercially prepared from lignin, a polymer of unknown chemical structure which is similar to coniferyl alcohol. Wood contains about 25 to 30 percent lignin and sulfite waste liquors up to 6 percent. In 1967, the Crown Zellerbach Paper Company obtained a patent for the processing of this black-liquor waste. The process utilized the methyl groups of kraft lignin by adding molten sulfur to form dimethyl sulfide. Nitrogen tetroxide was then used to oxidize the dimethyl sulfide into dimethyl sulfoxide. DMSO is inexpensive to produce, contrary to the excessive

**Source of commercial preparation**

prices charged by some of the pharmaceutical purveyors.

**Solvent capabilities**

DMSO is used commercially as a solvent for acetylene, sulfur dioxide, and other gases. It will dissolve most aromatic and unsaturated hydrocarbons, organic nitrogen compounds, organo-sulfur compounds, and many inorganic salts. It is used as a paint and varnish remover and is a solvent for Orlon, a polyacrylontrile fiber. DMSO is also used as an antifreeze and hydraulic fluid when mixed with water.

**Stability**

DMSO is stable up to 100°C in alkaline, acidic, or neutral conditions. It is stable at temperatures approaching its boiling point of 189°C in neutral or alkaline conditions. DMSO can be distilled away from solid caustic at atmospheric pressure. It can undergo slow decomposition under prolonged refluxing at atmospheric pressure. The rate of decomposition is a time-temperature function that can be accelerated by the addition of acids and retarded by bases.

**Reaction solvent**

DMSO is valuable as a reaction solvent for displacement, elimination and condensation reactions involving anions. The known reactions of DMSO have produced a variety of interesting compounds which have offered new avenues for synthesizing industrial materials (Crown Zellerbach, 1980). Aside from the varied industrial applications of DMSO, it has also displayed an equally fascinating array of therapeutic uses in the field of medicine.

**Trade names**

DMSO is sold under various trade names including: SQ9453, DMS-70, DMS-90, Deltan, Demasorb, Demavet, Demso, Dermasorb, Dolicur, Domoso, Dromisol, Gamasol 90, Hyadur, Infiltrina, Somipront, Syntexan, Topsyn, etc.

**Molecular structure**

The DMSO molecule is a tetrahedron, the center of which is occupied by a sulfur atom; two methyl groups, an oxygen atom and a nonbonding electron paid, are located at each apex (Fig. 1). The empirical formula of DMSO is $C_2H_6OS$. The molecular weight is 78.13. It has an elemental composition of C 30.74 percent, H 7.4 percent, O 20.48 percent, S 41.03 percent. Some of the physical properties of DMSO are given in Table I.

**Odor, taste, color**

DMSO is a very hygroscopic liquid and in pure form has practically no odor or color. It has a slightly bitter taste with a sweet after-taste.

**Dipolar aprotic solvent**

DMSO is a dipolar aprotic solvent. Protic solvents, such as water, methanol, and formamide, are hydrogen donors. Dipolar aprotic solvents, such as acetone, nitrobenzene, sulfur dioxide, and DMSO, lack the ability to donate labile hydrogen atoms, even though they possess hydrogen atoms, to form strong hydrogen bonds with other substances. DMSO tends to accept rather than donate protons.

**Ionic state**

DMSO in pure form is highly associated and possesses an ordered structure. This association is thermolabile at temperatures between 40 to 60°C. In its polarized form (Fig. 1), both the oxygen and sulfur of DMSO have unshared electron pairs. When DMSO is in its ionic form, it is able to dissolve salts or other ionic substances. The presence of three sets of unpaired electrons on the oxygen atom enable it to function as an electron donor (base) in complex formation with other substances.

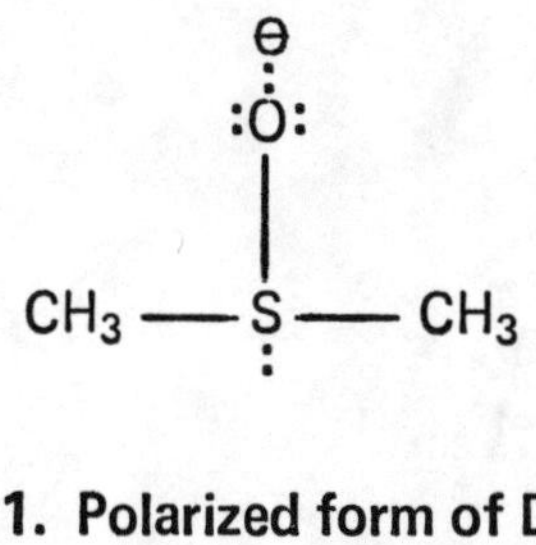

**Figure 1. Polarized form of DMSO**

# TABLE I

## Physical Properties of DMSO (from Szmant, 1971)

| PROPERTY | VALUE |
|---|---|
| Boiling point at 760 mm Hg, °C | 189.0 |
| Vapor pressure at 20°C, mm Hg | 0.37, 0.417 |
| Specific heat at 25°C, cal/g | 0.4698 |
| Specific heat of vaporization at b.p., cal/g | 175 |
| Molar heat of vaporization at b.p., kcal/mole | 13.67 |
| Entropy of vaporization at b.p., cal/deg. mole | 29.6 |
| Enthalpy of vaporization at 25°C, kcal/mole | 12.64 |
| Coefficient of expansion, ml/g. deg | 0.00088 |
| Specific gravity at 25°C, g/ml | 1.0958 |
| | 1.095566 |
| Melting point, °C | 18.55 |
| Specific heat of fusion, cal/g | 38.8 |
| Molar heat of fusion, kcal/mole | 3.43 |
| | 3.03 |
| Entropy of fusion, cal/deg. mole | 10.4 |
| | 11.7 |
| Specific heat of solid at 18.45°C, cal/g | 0.5 |
| Heat of formation (graphite and $S_{rhomb.}$), kcal/mole | –47.7 |
| Heat of combustion, cal/g | 6050 |
| Flash point, open vessel, °C | 95 |
| Molal f.p. depression, deg/mole/1000 g | 4.4, 4.36 |
| Refractive index ($n_D^{20}$) | 1.4783 |
| Refractive index ($n_D^{25}$) | 1.47674 |
| Molar refractivity, $R_m$ | 20.12 |
| Polarizability, $cm^3$ | $7.97 \times 10^{-24}$ |
| Dielectric constant at 20°C | 48.9 |
| Dielectric constant at 25°C | 46.4 |
| Dipole moment, 25°C, D | 4.11 |
| Viscosity, 20°C, cP | 2.473 |
| Viscosity, 25°C, cp | 1.99 |
| Surface tension at 20°C, dyne/cm | 46.2 |
| Surface tension at 25°C, dyne/cm | 42.86 |
| Specific conductance at 20°C, $ohm^{-1}$ $cm^{-1}$ | $3 \times 10^{-8}$ |

**Solvent characteristics**

The broad solvent characteristics of DMSO are the result of its ability to form either stable solvates by dipole-dipole interactions or solvent-solute associations by hydrophobic interactions. The marked polarity of the S-O bond is responsible for the high dielectric constant of DMSO in the liquid state. As a result of the dipole-dipole attractions of the S-O dipole, the molecules of DMSO are held together in the liquid state in a chain-like order.

**Molecular bonding with water**

DMSO is extremely hygroscopic and miscible with water in all proportions. The hygroscopic properties of DMSO explain some of the biological activities that are induced by this solvent. It is noteworthy that the hydrogen bonds which exist between water and DMSO are stronger than the hydrogen bonds which exist between water molecules (Cowie and Toporowski, 1961; Rammler and Zaffaroni, 1967). It is this hydrogen bonding activity of DMSO with water molecules and the greater activity of its anionic oxygen atom which differentiates DMSO from other aprotic solvents.

**Basicity**

The enhanced electron density at the oxygen atom contributes to the basicity of DMSO, which is slightly greater than that of water. DMSO forms crystalline salts with strong aprotic acids and coordinates with Lewis acids. DMSO tends to participate as the acceptor atom in hydrogen bonding. The ability of DMSO to compete effectively for hydrogen donor molecules is an important factor in the effect of DMSO in some of its chemical reaction rates.

**Chelating agent**

DMSO acts as a chelating agent. DMSO solvates cation because of the enhanced electron density at the oxygen atom and the steric availability of the oxygen. The DMSO ligand is almost always attached to the cation through the oxygen (Mac Gregor, 1967).

The unique molecular structure of DMSO and the

**Diversity of biological effects**

diversity of related structures it is able to form accounts for the wide variety of biological and therapeutic effects resulting from the use of this substance.

**Membrane penetrability**

One of the remarkable features of DMSO is its ability to cross the skin barrier rapidly and in high concentrations. Moreover, this feat is accomplished with little or no permanent tissue damage. This unique ability of membrane penetrability sets DMSO apart from all other solvents. The innocuous passage of DMSO through a protein barrier is believed to be the result of reversible configurational changes of proteins. This is due to the substitution of water by DMSO which causes a "loosening" of the protein structure. There may also be changes in enzymatic activity due to the action of DMSO by a variety of mechanisms which at present are not completely understood. The major configurational changes of the proteins occurs with DMSO concentrations of 60 to 70 volume percent (Hamaguchi, 1964). When the DMSO is removed, the configurational changes of the protein reverse to their normal structure.

**Configurational changes**

The cellular alterations by DMSO have been explained on the basis of its capacity to substitute for, or bind, water and the effects of DMSO on other hydrogen-bonded structures. The principal chemical constituent of the cell is water. The cellular biopolymers, such as proteins, polysaccharides, and nucleic acids, are surrounded by ordered arrays of water molecules sometimes referred to as the "hydration sheath" or bound water. Cellular structures are dependent upon this bound water, plus hydrophobic interactions, hydrogen bonds, and other stabilizing forces. Substitution or removal of the hydration sheath of these substances alters their configuration. The reverse of this process occurs either by diffusion or active transport of the major amount of DMSO from the tissues and gradual removal of the protein-bound DMSO by competitive bonding with cellular water.

**Affinity for water**

Studies of subunit proteins have also suggested that

the association of subunits is often stabilized not only by hydrogen bonding and hydrophobic bonding, but also by bound water and water bridges between proton-donor and proton-acceptor groups on a surface of the proteins. It was found that exposure of subunit proteins to low DMSO levels results in reversible alterations in protein structure, but there may be irreversible denaturation of subunit proteins at higher DMSO concentrations (Henderson, Henderson, and York, 1975).

**Alterations in protein structure**

The substitution and binding properties of DMSO probably account for its ability to assist in the therapeutic clearing of inflammatory conditions in the body.

**Effect on inflammatory conditions**

DMSO has radioprotective properties. However, the exact mechanism involved is not completely understood. DMSO has been found to protect the enzymes catalase and lactic acid dehydrogenase when exposed to x-rays. Since both of these enzymes contain metal ions (Fe in catalase and Zn in dehydrogenase), it has been suggested that the radioprotective properties of DMSO are based on its ability to scavenge free radicals (Roubal and Tappel, 1966). It is probable that DMSO protects against the lethal effects of whole-body radiation through several mechanisms, the full nature of which is not understood (Ashwood-Smith, 1971).

**Radioprotective properties**

DMSO has also been shown to have cryoprotective properties. The ability of DMSO to protect tissues at low temperatures has been explained on the basis of its colligative properties. Thus, DMSO lowers the concentration of electrolytes in equilibrium with ice at any temperature below freezing. If sufficient DMSO is present, the electrolyte concentration does not rise to a critically damaging level until the temperature is so low that the damage produced by the increased electrolyte level is reduced sufficiently to be tolerated by the cell (Ashwood-Smith, 1971).

**Cryoprotective properties**

DMSO may influence the chemical activity of enzyme systems. DMSO generally tends to stimulate enzymatic

**DMSO and enzymatic activity**

activity. It may change the substrate specificity of enzymes. This may occur by DMSO binding itself to certain groups at the active site thereby modifying substrate acceptance and rejection. Studies with lysozyme have shown that DMSO caused measureable changes in protein conformation. It appears that enzymes can function in high concentrations of DMSO with little loss of activity (Rammler, 1971).

**Effect on catecholamines**

The dipolar solvent characteristics of DMSO appear to facilitate the entry of catecholamines (dopamine, norepinephrine, and epinephrine) across the blood-brain barrier. It has been suggested that this phenomenon may be related to the ability of DMSO to serve as a carrier of biogenic amines to traverse both aqueous and lipid phases of components of the barrier (Hanig, Morrison, and Krop, 1971).

**Effect on nucleic acids**

DMSO in high concentrations is extremely effective in destabilizing the secondary structure of nucleic acids. It is believed that this destabilization is the result of the disruption of hydrophobic interactions between purine and/or pyrimidine bases (Rammler, 1971).

**Cellular immunity**

Studies have also been conducted on the influence of DMSO on cellular immunity. It was found that DMSO in conjunction with phytohemagglutin (PHA) increased the incorporation of tritiated thymidine and the production of interferon by lymphocytes of patients with chronic lymphatic leukemia over that induced by PHA or DMSO alone (Bartfield and Goldstein, 1975).

**Effects on prostaglandin synthesis**

DMSO stimulates the synthesis of prostaglandin $E_1$. Prostaglandins are a group of naturally occurring, chemically-related, long-chain hydroxy fatty acids that have a wide range of biological effects in the body. Essential fatty acids are necessary precursors of prostaglandins. Prostaglandins have biological activities of a hormonal and regulatory nature, and among other things, affect smooth muscle contractibility. The prostaglandins are named according to their ring substituents and the number of additional side-chain double bonds which have the cis configuration. The best known prostaglandins are $E_1$, $F_1$, and $F_2$. However, a large number of prostaglandins are known and new ones are being discovered periodically. In the lung, the E series prostaglandins are vasodilators and bronchodilators, whereas the F series are vasoconstrictors and bronchoconstrictors. It is believed by some investigators that one of the factors in the causation of asthma is an imbalance in the ratio of these two series of prostaglandins. If this hypothesis is correct, the fact that DMSO stimulates prostaglandin $E_1$ may be the reason why it is useful in the treatment of some cases of asthma.

**Metabolism of DMSO**

In the course of metabolism, DMSO is reduced to dimethyl sulfide and dimethyl sulfone (Rammler and Zaffaroni, 1967; Distefano and Borgstedt, 1964; Williams, et. al., 1965).

**Chemical references**

The chemistry of DMSO is extremely complex and is still in the process of evaluation. The foregoing resume touches on only a few of the many and diversified aspects of this remarkable agent. For further information on this subject, see the chemical reports by Distefano and Borgstedt (1964), Williams, et. al. (1965), Kharasch and Thyagarajan (1966), Hucker, et. al. (1967), Porter and Brey (1967), Rammler and Zaffaroni (1967), Mac Gregor (1967), Sweat and Epstein (1967), Rammler (1971), Embry and Dungard (1971), Hanig, Morrison, and Krop (1971), Ashwood-Smith (1971), Szmant (1971), David (1972), Hamar, Huang, and Chow (1974), Robinson (1975), Bartfield and Goldstein (1975), Misch and Misch (1975), Sandborn, Stephens, and Bendayan (1975), Henderson, Henderson, and York (1975), Ashwood-Smith (1975), Wood and Wood (1975), Conover (1975), Szmant (1975), LaHann and Horita (1975), Merck Index (1976), Crown Zellerbach (1980).

# 3

# How It Works

Dimethyl sulfoxide has the broadest pharmacological action of any known chemical agent. Jacob (1980) has suggested that it should be reviewed as a "therapeutic principle" rather than merely a "drug." A drug is a substance that influences certain diseases, whereas DMSO therapy is, in reality, a new way of treating a disease process. The pharmacological properties of DMSO are varied and suggest new approaches to certain disease therapies.

**DMSO as a "therapeutic principle"**

In a sense, DMSO seems to possess some of the characteristics of what Soviet scientists have referred to as an adaptogenic substance, i.e., a substance that produces a normalizing effect on the body.

**Adaptogen**

One of the more phenomenal and unique actions of DMSO is its ability to cross most membranes of the body without destroying membrane integrity. In its passage through membranes, DMSO has the ability to carry with it a number of other chemical agents. This membrane penetration phenomenon is reversible. Tooth enamel and nails are essentially the only body tissues that are impervious to DMSO.

**Membrane penetrability**

Studies on the membrane penetration and transport effects of DMSO have been carried out in plants, lower animals, and man. The pioneer study by Jacob, Bischel, and Herschler (1964) demonstrated the penetration and transport capacity of DMSO across the mucous membrane of dog bladders. Kolb, et. al. (1967) found radioactive DMSO in blood samples within five minutes of skin application.

**Transport of substances through membranes by DMSO**

There have been numerous studies on the ability of DMSO to carry various other substances with it through biological membranes. It has been found that nonionized molecules of low molecular weight pass through membrane barriers with the greatest ease. DMSO will carry hydrogen peroxide into the myocardium of the heart (Finney, et. al., 1967), and will carry antibodies to serum albumin through rabbit skin (Jacob, 1969). Maddock, Green, and Brown (1966) showed the ability of DMSO to carry antitumor agents. Further studies concluded that there was a threefold increase in dermal penetration of testosterone and hydrocortisone when they were dissolved in DMSO (Mailbach and Feldmann, 1967) and that penicillin was readily carried through intact human skin (Perlman and Wolfe, 1966). A very remarkable phenomenon of DMSO is its ability to pass through the blood-brain barrier *in vivo* (Brink and Stein, 1967; de la Torre, 1970). There are many other in-depth studies on the ability of DMSO to transport other substances through membrane barriers that will not be discussed, but are reviewed by Stoughton and Fritsch (1964), Horrita and Weber (1964), Kligman (1965), Skog and Wahlberg (1967), Baker (1968), David (1972), Astley and Levine (1975).

The mechanism of the increased membrane permeability and transport of DMSO is not completely known. However, it is thought that the rapid movement of DMSO through the skin, a protein barrier, is dependent on a reversible configurational change of the protein that occurs when DMSO substitutes for water. DMSO has a strong attraction to water. See section on Chemistry for further details (pp. 27-28).

In laboratory studies, DMSO exerted a significant effect on lessening the edema produced in rats paws following induced tissue injury and injection of autologous blood. Topical DMSO application reduced both of these types of edema (Formanek and Kovak, 1966). Carageenin-induced paw edema was decreased by oral and topical DMSO therapy. Arthritis induced in rats was found to be inhibited by DMSO (Gorog and Kovacs, 1968). In guinea pigs, DMSO was found to exhibit anti-inflammatory activity against Baker's yeast granuloma (Jacob, 1969).

**Anti-inflammatory activity**

In understanding the anti-inflammatory effect of DMSO, Weisman, Sessa, and Bevans (1967) found that lysosomes can be stabilized with cortisone against a variety of injurious agents. The concentration of these agents necessary to stabilize lysosomes is reduced from 10 to 1,000 fold when dissolved in DMSO. It is probably that DMSO renders steroids more available to their targets within tissues.

**Analgesic activity**

It appears that pain relief from the topical administration of DMSO to affected areas involves more than anti-inflammatory action, vasodilitation, or local analgesia. Dermal application of DMSO a distance from the affected area produces relief from pain and inflammation which suggests DMSO depresses the central nervous system pain center or has been carried by the blood to the affected area, or both. Perhaps the analgesic effect is produced by the depression of nerve conduction from the affected area (David, 1972).

**Effects on neuromuscular transmission**

Gandiha and Marshall (1972) observed that DMSO affects neuromuscular transmission. They found DMSO exerts a direct depressant action on cholinesterase activity and on skeletal muscle. It produces greater action on neurally-stimulated preparations than on directly-stimulated preparations. This may indicate that DMSO possesses additional actions on the process of neuromuscular transmission. DMSO was found to cause repression of reactive capacities of hemoreceptors. These actions cease very rapidly after the termination of DMSO therapy (Litvinchuk and Nevelichuk, 1972).

**Nerve conduction**

Young, et. al. (1968) found that when DMSO was applied directly to a peripheral sensory nerve, it directly blocked nerve conduction in the smallest C fibers. When application was continued, it progressively and differentially blocked fibers from small to large, depending on the length of time it was applied.

Sciatic nerve immersion in 6 percent DMSO was found to decrease the nerve conduction velocity by 40 percent. Washing the nerve in a buffer for one hour totally reversed this effect (Sams, 1967).

**Effects on pain**

Subcutaneous injections of 10 percent DMSO in cats induced a total loss of central pain response. Two ml of 50 percent DMSO injected into the cerebrospinal fluid produced total anesthesia in the animal for thirty minutes. Complete recovery occurred following the experiment (Jacob, 1971).

**Anesthesia**

Dermal anesthesia in humans was obtained by topical application of a 2 percent concentration of tetracaine base combined with 100 percent DMSO. This anesthetic effect was intense and unquestionable (Brechner, et. al., 1967).

**Bacteriostasis**

DMSO has been found to exert a marked inhibitory effect on a wide range of fungi and bacteria, including at least one parasite, at concentrations of 30 to 50 percent. Jacob, et. al. (1964) found 20 percent DMSO to be bacteriostatic against *Escherichia coli*, *Staphylococcus aureus*, and *Pseudomonas* and in 5 percent concentration, bacteriostatic against tubercle bacillus. Aqueous solutions of 35 percent and higher are self-sterilizing. Jacob and Wood (1967) mention the studies of Tsuchiya, Iriyama, and Umezaua (1964) who suggest the antibacterial effect results from the production of methylmethanthiosulfinate from DMSO. DMSO may interfere with bacterial growth by altering the RNA conformation structure that is required for protein synthesis.

DMSO in 12.5 to 25 percent concentrations was found to cause complete inhibition of growth of high pleomorphic bacteria regularly isolated from human leukemic bloods and tumors. This growth inhibition was obtained in all twenty-seven isolated organisms without adverse effects on the intact red blood cells (Seibert, et. al., 1967).

**Effects on antibiotic sensitivity**

Jacob and Wood further cited a study conducted by Kamiya, et. al. (1966) who evaluated the effect of 5 percent DMSO on the increased sensitivity of bacteria to antibiotics. They found DMSO increased and restored the sensitivity of antibiotic-resistant strains. Sensitivity restoration was obtained in some strains of *E. coli* and *Psuedomonas.* Antibiotics not effective on certain bacteria showed growth-inhibitory effects when combined with DMSO. DMSO was effective in overcoming streptomycin resistance in *E. coli.*

**Diuresis**

Urine output resulting from systemic or dermal administration of DMSO depends on the total amount of DMSO given, not the degree of dilution reached. It appears that DMSO exerts an osmotic diuretic action (DiStefano and Klahn, 1965).

DMSO was administered topically to rats in a dosage of 0.5ml of 90 percent solution repeated five times daily. Urine volume increased tenfold. Sodium and potassium excretion showed an increase as well. Similar results were obtained with oral DMSO (Formanek and Suckert, 1966).

**Drug enhancement**

DMSO has been found to enhance the activity of other compounds dissolved in it. This action is thought to be related to increased membrane penetration. It synergizes blood sugar depression when DMSO and insulin are given intravenously to dogs. It increases the anti-inflammatory effect of cortisone (Jacob, 1965).

Mellville and colleagues (1968) found that DMSO enhances the action of digitoxin on the heart in cats without degradation of the glycoside or involving myocardial fixation.

**Effects on toxicity**

In toxicity studies conducted on animals, the $LD_{50}$ (lethal dose of half of the subjects) was calculated on drugs combined with DMSO. Toxicity of pentolinium tartrate and hexamethonium bitartrate was increased by DMSO, while toxicity of hexamethonium iodide was decreased. The reduction in effectiveness may be secondary to inactivation of the dissolved compound by DMSO (Rosen, et. al., 1965).

**Immune response**

In a study on antigen antibody reactions it was found that DMSO did not disturb the immune response. Oral administration of DMSO to animals for ten days prior to an infection with murine typhus enhanced resistance to the infection and produced leukocytosis (Raettig, 1966).

Kunze (1975) found DMSO increased interferon titers 2 to 16 fold in mice infected with Calova and Sindkis viruses.

Collagen deposition takes place in the formation of intestinal adhesions, inflammatory repair process, and in scleroderma.

**Collagen deposition**

In skin biopsy specimens taken from scleroderma patients prior to treatment with DMSO and at three-week intervals, a dissolution of collagen was found while the elastic fibers remained intact (Scherbel, et. al., 1967). DMSO exerts a significant effect on pathological deposition of collagen in postirradiation subcutaneous fibrosis in humans, but it does not appear to alter collagen metabolism equilibrium in normal tissue (Gries, et. al., 1967). Keloids, more commonly known as scars, that were biopsied prior to and following DMSO therapy showed a histological improvement towards normalcy (Engel, 1967).

**Collagen destruction**

It is not clear whether DMSO initiates abnormal collagen destruction and eventual disappearance or whether it merely increases cellular permeability which allows for the release of proteolytic enzymes. It appears that the biochemical reaction responsible for histologic changes in collagen is selective for collagen (Jacob, 1965).

**Histamine-liberation properties**

DMSO possesses a potent histamine-liberating property at the site of dermal application which results in increased blood flow to the skin (Kligman, 1965). A study was conducted on pedicle flaps on the backs of rats that had length to width ratios of three to one. Topical application of 70 percent DMSO three times daily decreased the anticipated skin slough by 60 to 70 percent. Photomicrographs taken by Adamson and colleagues (1966) indicated blood vessel dilitation beneath the skin of rabbit ears treated topically with DMSO.

**Myocardial lesions**

Jacob (1971) noted that DMSO therapy for myocardial lesions in animals reduced residual myocardial fibrosis and effected a distinct modification with a decrease in myocardial fiber necrosis. There were no aneurysms or myocardial ruptures in the group of animals treated with DMSO.

**Effects on muscles and nerves**

Sams (1967) evaluated cardiac, skeletal, and smooth muscle reaction to concentrations of 0.6 to 6 percent DMSO. He found that DMSO markedly depressed response of the diaphragm to direct (muscle) and indirect (nerve) electrical stimulation and led to production of spontaneous fisciculations of the skeletal muscle. However, he found the response of the smooth muscle of the stomach to muscle and nerve stimulation was increased by DMSO. A 6 percent solution of DMSO lowered the vagal threshold by 50 percent. An *in vitro* assay study concluded that 0.8 to 8 percent DMSO inhibited bovine erythrocyte cholinesterase 16 to 85 percent, respectively (Sams, et. al., 1966).

**Muscle relaxation**

DMSO applied topically to the skin of patients suffering muscle spasms produced electromyographic evidence of muscle relaxation one hour following application (Birkmayer, et. al., 1966).

**Effects on platelets**

A 5 percent solution of DMSO was found to lessen the adhesiveness of blood platelets *in vitro* (Deutsch and Kock, 1966). A laboratory test on hamsters also showed DMSO to be a useful antagonist against thrombus formation and platelet aggregation *in vivo* (Jacob, 1971).

**Effects on cholesterol**

A clinical trial was conducted on rabbits given a high cholesterol diet containing 1 percent DMSO. The DMSO-treated animals had only one half the hypercholesteremia of the control group (Herzmann, 1968).

**Radioprotective effects**

The mechanism of the radioprotective action of DMSO is not fully understood, although several experiments indicate it is a cellular rather than an indirect pharmacological mechanism. See section on Chemistry (p. 30) for further details. DMSO may be involved in modifying effects that interfere with the hydrogen bonding process. This protective action can operate in systems that vary from bacterial cells and enzymes to tissue culture cells and whole animals (Ashwood-Smith, 1971, 1975).

**Effects on enzymes**

At the molecular level, DMSO protects the enzymes catalase and lactic acid dehydrogenase from inactivation by radiation. It could be that DMSO metal ion-enzyme complexes are involved in radioprotection (Lohmann and Moss, 1966).

**X-ray dosage**

Dermal application of 30 percent DMSO to 16-day-old rats for twenty minutes prior to x-irradiation protected them against x-ray induced damage (Dodd and Sherwell, 1968). Mice were completely protected from cataract induction by a dosage of 1,000 radians of x-rays when DMSO was topically applied to the eyes prior to treatment (Hagemann, et. al., 1970). Intra-abdominal administration of DMSO to *Drosophila melanogaster* was found to significantly reduce sex-linked recessive lethal mutation of male sperm, the frequency of II-III translocations induced by x-rays to male sperm, and x-ray-induced mortality (Barnett, 1972).

**Treatment with DMSO**

Kim and Moos (1966) found that topical application of DMSO to rats prior to radiation exposure provided considerable protection. The animals receiving DMSO experienced less weight loss than the control group. Treatment with

DMSO after irradiation had no effect on mortality. A study conducted by Ashwood-Smith (1967) showed that DMSO protected 70 percent of the mice from radiation death. There were no survivors in the control group.

**Cryoprotection**

It is very likely that the cryoprotective and radioprotective actions of DMSO are closely related. The concept originally proposed by Lovelock and Bishop (1959) is that DMSO has the ability to lower the concentration of electrolytes in equilibrium with ice at any temperature that is below freezing. Nash (1966) found that the most important property possessed by an effective endocellular cryophylactic agent such as DMSO is the strong affinity it possesses for water.

It has been indicated by Meryman (1971) that DMSO functions on a colligative basis in permeating the cells. Litvan (1972) concluded that the cryoprotective action is induced by the diminution of both the migration rate of water and vapor pressure difference between extracellular ice and interacellular water.

In aqueous solution, DMSO prevents the crystalline formation of ice within frozen red blood cells. Migration of ice crystals during the thawing process results in cell death through a disruption of structural elements. DMSO at concentrations between 5 to 10 percent appears to be the best cryoprotective agent for mammalian cell systems. Cooling rates between 1° and 20° C/minute and thawing rates of 100° C/minute enable between 50 to 95 percent of the cells to survive. DMSO has been found to be superior over glycerol as a cryoprotective agent. Because it can penetrate cells with ease and decrease osmotic insult, it is used as a preservative for spermatozoa, bacteria, bone marrow, blood tissue culture cells, and trypanosomes (Ashwood-Smith, 1975; Graham, 1975).

Studies conducted on animals (de la Torre and Rowed, 1974) indicated that DMSO stimulated respiration and protected against anoxic stress. It appeared such stimulation was central in origin. Tests found that rats exposed to inhalation of pure nitrogen gas were protected from hypoxic death by DMSO. Walker and associates (1966) found that DMSO reduces the rate of oxygen consumption in animals.

**Absorption**

*Absorption:* The rate of dermal absorption by DMSO is dependent on its concentration. An increasing rate of absorption is seen up to about 90 percent strength. The optimal concentration for absorption through the skin barrier is 70 to 90 percent.

When DMSO is applied to other membranes, lower concentrations can be employed. Excellent tissue penetration is obtained in the bladder with only a 15 percent aqueous solution (Herschler and Jacob, 1980).

Kolb, et. al. (1967) studied the rapidity of the appearance of topically applied DMSO in the blood of the rat, dog, and man using sulfur-35 and radio-labeled DMSO. The DMSO was detected in the blood of man at five minutes when the first sample was drawn. A maximal level was reached within four to six hours and remained at a plateau for 1.5 to 3 days. Similar studies (Hucker, et. al., 1965, 1966, 1967) reported rapid cutaneous absorption in man with peak levels after four to eight hours. It was detected in blood serum for as long as 400 hours following application. After oral and intraperitoneal administration, peak levels were found within one-half to one hour of treatment. In six hours, half the peak blood level was gone and only 5 to 10 percent remained 24 hours after administration. DMSO was undetectable after 120 hours.

**Distribution studies**

*Distribution:* Distribution studies conducted on laboratory animals one hour after dermal application found labeled DMSO throughout the body including all bones and connective tissue (Kolb, et. al., 1967). Topical radio-labeled DMSO was noted to rapidly accumulate in both soft and hard tissues (Denko, et. al., 1967). Ashwood-Smith (1961) observed a rapid accumulation of labeled DMSO in blood, spleen, testes, liver, kidney, and brain. The highest concentrations were found in the kidney and the lowest in the lung in a study conducted by McDermot and colleagues (1967).

**Bio-transformation**

*Biotransformation:* The metabolites of DMSO are dimethyl sulfide (DMSO) and dimethyl sulfone ($DMSO_2$). Failure to identify metabolic products other than DMS and $DMSO_2$ indicates that a simple oxidation-reduction system exists. This is not the case in microorganisms, however, because they are capable of metabolizing the entire DMSO molecule (Wood, 1971).

**Excretion**

*Excretion:* In man, cutaneous administration of DMSO $^{35}$–S showed that it was completely excreted within 48 hours. $DMSO_2$ was noted eight hours after treatment and continued to be excreted for 480 hours (Hucker, et. al., 1965, 1966). Thirteen percent was excreted in the urine as DMSO and 18 percent as $DMSO_2$. The urine recovery of DMSO following oral administration was 50.8 percent and 22 percent for $DMSO_2$. After intravenous administration in man, 80 percent of the original dose of DMSO was recovered within eight days. The kidney is the major organ of excretion. Man excretes little DMSO in the feces (Kolb, et. al., 1965, 1966).

**Pharmacology references**

Excellent reviews on the pharmacology of DMSO have been written by Jacob, et. al. (1964), Block (1964), Farrant (1964), Distefano and Klahn (1965), Jacob (1965), Kolb, et. al. (1965), Rosen, et. al. (1965), Kligman (1965), McDermot, et. al. (1967), Bradham and Sample (1967), Jacob and Wood (1967), Kolb, et. al. (1967), Ashwood-Smith (1967), Young, et. al. (1968), Jacob (1969), Jacob and Wood (1971), Ashwood-Smith (1971), Jacob (1971), David (1972), Litvinchuk and Nevelichuk (1972), Spiker (1972), Gandiha and Marshall (1972), Wood and Wood (1975), Kocsis, et. al. (1975), Ashwood-Smith (1975), Herschler and Jacob (1980).

# 4

# Is It Safe?

The science dealing with poisons or toxins is known as toxicology. Untoward effects are produced by drugs because of their toxicity. The term toxicity to the non-professional is frequently interpreted to mean any substance which, when ingested or injected, is likely to produce death or some sort of a severe reaction. This interpretation is only partially correct. Foods, drugs, and poisons have one thing in common: each of them is capable of producing some sort of a biological effect. The effects of most foods to most people tend to be relatively mild in nature. In the case of drugs, the effects are generally more pronounced and predictable in the sense that their toxic range is largely controlled by established dosage levels. Poisons tend to be more violent since their dosage range, particularly when encountered accidentally, is uncontrolled. Nevertheless, it should be noted that on occasion, foods, drugs, and poisons may produce serious unexpected side effects. The range of reactions of even an essential nutrient may vary from a lethal deficiency state, to a moderate deficiency state, to optimum health, to a toxic level, or lethality, as the dosage is increased. This

**Toxicology defined**

**Dose response**

toxicological principle is best stated in a dictum expressed by the famous Swiss physician Theophrastus Paracelsus who lived during the period from 1493 to 1541, namely: "All substances are poisons; there is none which is not a poison. The right dose differentiates a poison from a remedy." This is the reason why a precise definition is difficult to formulate because it includes virtually every known chemical and physical agent, depending upon the exact conditions of exposure. A poison produces harm only within prescribed conditions of usage. DMSO is no different than any other chemical substance; its toxic effects are governed by these fundamental toxicological principles.

**So-called "dangers" of DMSO**

The FDA has made exaggerated claims concerning the toxic effects of DMSO on man. However, their claims have little basis in human toxicological reality. Therefore, it is important that the patient be fully informed as to the scientific facts concerning the so-called "dangers" of using DMSO.

In order to understand the following discussion on the toxicity of DMSO, it is necessary to define some of the terms that are used in toxicology.

**Toxic substance defined**

*Toxic Substance:* A toxic substance is one that demonstrates the potential to induce cancer, tumors, or neoplastic effects in human or experiemental animals; to induce a permanent transmissible change in the characteristics of an offspring from those of its human or experimental animal parents; to cause the production of physical defects in the developing human or experimental animal embryo; to produce death in experimental or domestic animals exposed via the respiratory tract, skin, eye, mouth, or other routes; to produce irritation or sensitization of the skin, eyes, or respiratory passages; to diminish mental alertness, reduce motivation, or alter behavior of humans; to adversely affect the health of a normal or disabled person of any age or of either sex by producing reversible or irreversible bodily injury or by endangering life or causing death from exposure via the respiratory tract, skin, eye, mouth, or any other route in any quantity, concentration, or dose reported for any length of time.

**Lethal response,**

*Lethal Response:* The death of the organism in response to single or short-term exposures to toxic substances is usually given because it is the most definitive toxicity data generally provided by toxicologists. However, the acute or immediate toxic effect does not necessarily characterize the toxicity of those substances for which other effects may predominate, such as cumulative effects from longer term exposure.

**$LD_{50}$**

*$LD_{50}$ (Lethal Dose Fifty):* A calculated dose of a chemical substance which is expected to cause the death of fifty percent of an entire defined experimental animal population, as determined from the exposure to the substance, by any route other than inhalation, of a significant number of animals from that population.

**Routes of administration**

*Route of Administration:* The toxic reactions to a substance generally varies according to the route of administration. When a substance is administered via the oral (mouth) route, there is usually a delay, and because of the gastrointestinal barrier, the animal may appear to tolerate a higher dosage than when administered by some other route. Parenteral administration, by some route other than the gastrointestinal tract, may result in varying rates of absorption and distribution of the poison throughout the body. The intravenous route results in an instantaneous accessibility to the circulating blood and the injected substance is rapidly distributed to every part of the body. The rapidity of absorption of most toxic substances from slowest to fastest is as follows: Topical, oral, intradermal, intramuscular, subcutaneous, intraperitoneal, inhalation, and intravenous. Generally, a dosage level that might be readily tolerated by the oral route may produce severe toxic reactions, or death, if that same dosage were given intravenously.

**Routes of administration defined**

*Oral (Mouth):* Administration of the toxic substance by the oral route.

*IP:* Administration of the toxic substance by the intraperitoneal route; the substance is injected into the abdominal cavity.

*IV:* Administration of the toxic substance intravenously, i.e., by injection into the vein.

**Mg/Kg defined**

*Mg/Kg (Milligram per Kilogram):* Refers to the milligrams of weight of the toxic substance per kilogram of weight of the test animal. This is a designation that is commonly used in toxicology since the dose response of an organism is generally related to its weight.

**Animal tests show low toxicity**

Most of our theoretical knowledge concerning the toxicity of any particular substance is derived from laboratory studies with animals. DMSO has now been studied extensively as to its effects in both laboratory mammals and humans. All of the studies, including the short and long-term administration of DMSO on fish, birds, a variety of laboratory mammals, and man, have consistently demonstrated that DMSO has a very low toxicity and is generally very well tolerated. However, in making generalizations of this type, one must always recognize the fact that no amount of experimental animal studies can guarantee absolute safety or efficacy to humans. Animal toxicity data does provide relative guidelines which have proved to be useful in establishing drug dosage levels in man. In evaluating drug toxicity it should be noted that the greater the dosage level, usually the safer the drug as far as acute toxicity is concerned. Table I will be helpful in interpreting the general toxicity dosage levels as given in Tables II and III later in this chapter. It is important to keep in mind that the effects on animals

**Animal studies no guarantee for human safety**

may vary with the species, dosage given, and the route of administration. There is also a great deal of biochemical individuality from one person to the next, all of which can result in variable responses in humans.

## TABLE II

### CLASSIFICATION OF RELATIVE TOXICITY CATEGORIES

| TOXICITY RATING | COMMONLY USED TERM | PROBABLY HUMAN LETHAL DOSE 70–kg (150–lb) MAN | |
|---|---|---|---|
| 6 | Supertoxic | < 5mg/kg | A taste–7 drops |
| 5 | Extremely toxic | 5-50mg/kg | 7 drops–1 teaspoonful |
| 4 | Very toxic | 50-500mg/kg | 1 tsp–1 ounce |
| 3 | Moderately toxic | 0.5-5g/kg | 1 oz–1 pint or pound |
| 2 | Slightly toxic | 5-15g/kg | 1 pint–1 quart |
| 1 | Practically nontoxic | > 15g/kg | 1 quart |

**General toxicity**

*General Toxicity:* The earliest studies on the toxicity of DMSO were published by Hixson (1955), Ashwood-Smith (1961), Brown, et. al. (1963), Rosenkratz, et. al (1963), and the more extensive work of Caujolle, et. al. (1957, 1964, 1965, 1967). There has since appeared a large number of scientific publications dealing with the acute and chronic toxic effects of DMSO. However, no attempt will be made to review all of these publications. The following is a resume of some of the more pertinent toxicological data as they relate to DMSO therapy in man.

## TABLE III
## TOXICITY OF DMSO ON LABORATORY ANIMALS
## SINGLE DOSE $LD_{50}$ (gm/km)

*(from Mason, 1971)*

| SPECIES | ROUTE OF ADMINISTRATION | | | | |
|---|---|---|---|---|---|
| | INTRAVENOUS | INTRAPERITONEAL | SUBCUTANEOUS | ORAL | DERMAL |
| Mouse | 3.8 – 8.9 | 14.6 – 20.6 | 13.9 – 25.6 | 16.5 – 24.6 | 44 |
| Rat | 5.2 – 8.1 | 5.5 – 13.6 | 13.7 | 17.4 – 28.3 | 40-50 |
| Rabbit | 6.0 – 8.0 | – | 14.0 | 14.0 | MDA* |
| Dog | 2.5 – 8.0 | – | – | 10.0 | MDA |
| Monkey | 4.0 – 8.0 | – | – | 4.0 | MDA |

*Maximum Dose Applicable

## TABLE IV
## COMPARATIVE DRUG TOXICITIES

| | COMMON DRUGS APPROVED BY THE FDA | | | | | | | |
|---|---|---|---|---|---|---|---|---|
| Test Animal | Actino-mycin D | Amphet-amine | Aspirin | Butazolidin | Digitalis | Inderal | Tetra cycline | Vitamin $B_1$ Thiamine |
| Oral Mouse | 13mg/kg | 45mg/kg | 815mg/kg | 630mg/kg | 3.5mg/kg | 471mg/kg | 808mg/kg | 8224mg/kg |
| IP Mouse | .07mg/kg | 23mg/kg | 495mg/kg | 100mg/kg | 5.5mg/kg | 125mg/kg | 125mg/kg | 220mg/kg |
| IV Mouse | .046mg/kg | 18mg/kg | 681mg/kg | 123mg/kg | 20mg/kg | 22mg/kg | 294mg/kg | 89mg/kg |

Areas of general concern to toxicologists include the amount of a drug that will cause lethality in fifty percent of the test animals ($LD_{50}$), which organs are primarily affected, and the dosage levels of the medication the test animal can tolerate.

**Areas of concern to toxicologists**

In attempting to evaluate the tolerance limits of DMSO, it is necessary to consider the various factors which influence these limits, viz.; (1) total amount of DMSO used; (2) rate of administration (single, multiple, slow or rapid); (3) route of administration (dermal, oral, intravenous, intramuscular, subcutaneous, etc.); (4) concentrations; (5) temperature (drug and recipient); (6) solubility or rate of release; (7) physical state (liquid, ointment, tablet, powder, capsule, etc.); (8) total volume administered; (9) excretion interference; (10) species variations; (11) age differences; (12) sex differences; (13) genetic enzyme differences; (14) induced enzymatic differences; (15) variations due to altered physiological or pathological conditions; (16) variations due to hypersensitivity or allergies. No attempt will be made to explore all of these factors since some of them go beyond the scope of this presentation, whereas others are difficult to assess because of the limitations of our knowledge. Nevertheless, these are parameters of the overall problem of toxicity that must be considered by both the patient and the physician.

**Factors which influence tolerance limits**

*Lethal Doses ($LD_{50}$'s) of DMSO:* It will be noted in Table II that there are some species differences in the $LD_{50}$'s of the various animals tested. The tests are based on the use of DMSO as a pure compound (100 percent). It will also be seen that since DMSO is of such a low order of toxicity that the $LD_{50}$'s are given in gm per kg of body weight rather than mg per kg as is the case in most other drugs. A comparison of the toxicity of DMSO can be made by examining some of the $LD_{50}$'s of other commonly used drugs that have been approved by the FDA as given in Table IV. DMSO is much safer to use than any of the other drugs listed, including aspirin, regardless of the route of administration.

**$LD_{50}$'s of DMSO**

**Low toxicity confirmed**

Although there are species differences as to modes and speeds of metabolism and excretion of DMSO, none of these factors have radically altered the overall view of low toxicity by whatever route of administration. It has been consistently observed that the ability of DMSO to be rapidly absorbed and spread throughout the body when taken orally or injected is so great that there is no evidence of increased toxicity with repeated daily administration of DMSO.

**Repeated doses found safe**

*Repeated Sublethal Doses:* DMSO does not accumulate in the tissues, consequently there is no typical delayed toxicity.

**Effects on blood vessels**

*Effects on Blood Vessels:* The effects on blood vessels varies according to the concentration of the DMSO being injected. The initial damage is very rapid and occurs when the concentration is above eighty percent. There may occur a perivascular inflammatory reaction when DMSO is given at high concentrations intravenously. The localized reaction may include intravascular thrombi with round cells, macrophages and plasma cell infiltration. No necrosis or sloughing takes place, and the original irritation and thrombi usually disappear within a short period of time. There may also be hemolysis and hemoglobinuria (Willson, et. al., 1965; Smith, et. al., 1967; Mason, 1971). At the dosage level DMSO is administered intravenously in most clinics, there are no untoward effects that have been observed.

**Local tissue reactions**

*Local Tissue Reactions:* Subcutaneous or intramuscular injections of DMSO may cause a localized hemorrhagic, gelatinous, or edematous reaction. The intensity of the reaction is proportional to the concentration and total amount of DMSO injected. No instances of abscess formation, necrosis, or sloughing have been reported (Rosenkrantz, et. al., 1963; Sommers and Tauberger, 1973; Smith, et. al., 1967, Mason, 1971).

**Effects on the liver**

*Liver:* The only cases in which liver damage has been observed are those in which high doses of DMSO have been injected into test animals. The liver damage consisted of degeneration of liver cells and inflammatory changes, hemolyzed red blood cells in the hapatic sinusoids and fragmentation of Kupfer cells (Rosenkratz, et. al., 1963; Willson, et. al., 1965; Shilkin, et. al., 1966; Caujolle, et. al., 1967; Wood, et. al., 1967; Mason, 1971).

**Effects on the kidneys**

*Kidney:* In test animals where high concentrations of DMSO have been injected, mild tubular nephrosis incidental to the breakdown of hemolysis products has been observed (Mason, 1971).

**Effects on the lungs**

*Lung:* Lung pathology has been observed in test animals which were given either lethal doses or after increasing higher doses of DMSO. In some of these cases, pulmonary edema was evidenced (Mason, 1971).

**Teratogenic effects**

The teratogenic effect of a substance is its tendency to induce the development of physical defects in offspring *in utero.* Teratogenic effects have been reported in rabbits, chickens, mice, and rats when they were administered very high dosages of DMSO (Caujolle, et. al., (1967). No teratogenic effects have been reported in humans.

**Cutaneous toxicity**

The application of DMSO to the skin is the route most commonly used in clinical medicine. The dermal route is the least toxic route of administration. DMSO passes rapidly through the skin and causes vasodilation and erythema in proportion to its concentration. The $LD_{50}$ of DMSO applied to the skin in mice is reported to be 44-50gm/kg which is an extremely low order of toxicity (Smith, et. al., 1968; Mason, 1971).

**Effects on the eyes**

**Changes in the refractive index observed**

It is generally believed that the possibility of damage to the lens of the eye is of primary toxicological significance in DMSO therapy. Reports from several investigators in the United States and England conducting chronic toxicity studies with DMSO in 1965 indicated that the drug caused changes in the refractive index of the eyes of certain laboratory animals, viz., dogs, rabbits, and swine. The Food and Drug

**FDA terminates testing**

Administration responded on November 25, 1965, in the Federal Register that "All exemptions for clinical testing of dimethylsulfoxide (DMSO) in man are hereby terminated effective on signature of this order (November 19, 1965). No person may ship dimethylsulfoxide (DMSO) within the jurisdiction of the Federal Food, Drug, and Cosmetic Act for clinical testing in man until this proposal has had advance approval by the Commissioner of Food and Drugs on the basis of a Notice of Claimed Investigational Exemption for a New Drug (form FD 1571) justifying such studies" (NAS, 1973).

**Kefauver-Harris Amendment**

The European thalidomide disaster in which numbers of infants were born with deformed limbs helped to precipitate the Kefauver-Harris Amendments to the Food and Drug Act on October 10, 1962, which supposedly was enacted to reinforce safety in the use of drugs. The thalidomide-Kefauver context has had a profound effect on the reticence of the FDA to approve the use of DMSO, according to some, whereas others attribute it to bureaucratic bungling. Regardless of the actual cause of the FDA's inactions, the subject of ocular toxicity remains a dominant issue in the entire DMSO matter. The FDA ban and the exaggerated claims regarding the dangers of using DMSO have generally caused the drug to fall into disrepute among American physicians. It is therefore important that the matter of ocular toxicity be discussed.

**Ocular toxicity discussed**

It was found that the administration of DMSO to certain laboratory animals could result in a selective alteration of the lens. The cortical fibers of the lens become less relucent than normal, but the relucency of the nucleus is undisturbed. This condition produces a refracting surface that is more convex than the lens surface, resulting in myopia. These eye changes have been found to occur in rabbits, swine, and dogs, but not monkeys. These eye changes have never been reported in man (Jacob, 1966; Jacob and Rosenbaum, 1966; Rubin and Mattis, 1966; Wolfred, 1966; Barnett and Noel, 1967; Caldwell, Bye, and Briggs, 1967; Caujolle, et. al., 1967; Gordon, 1967; Jacob and Wood, 1967; Petersen and Robertson, 1967; Smith, Hadidian, and Mason, 1967; Wood,

**Eye changes never reported in man**

et. al., 1967; Gordon and Kleberger, 1968; Fishman, et. al., 1969; Hull, Wood, and Brobyn, 1969; Smith, Mason, and Epstein, 1969; Vogin, et. al., 1970; Wood, Weber, and Palmquist, 1971; NAS, 1973; Brobyn, 1975; Rubin, 1975; Noel, et. al., 1975; Herschler and Jacob, 1980).

A study was conducted on the rate of absorption of DMSO when administered directly into the rat eye (Weaver, et. al., 1975). The results indicated that less than two percent of the dose is absorbed by the eye five minutes after application and 25 minutes later approximately 87 percent of the absorbed DMSO was cleared from the eye. The results revealed that the level of DMSO in the eye is in direct proportion to the concentration of DMSO applied.

**Tests to determine human ocular toxicity**

Several controlled studies have been conducted to ascertain the toxicity of DMSO in man. A study was conducted in New York (Gordon, 1967), where DMSO was administered at concentrations of 7.5 to 66 percent into the eyes of 108 patients over a period of one to fifteen months. There was no evidence of lens, cornea, or retina changes in the patients. Twenty-three of these patients had glaucoma or cataracts prior to treatment. During this time there was no evidence the DMSO aggravated their existing disorders.

Drs. Jacob and Rosenbaum of Oregon treated 32 patients for three to nineteen months with an average dose of 30 gm/day of DMSO (Brobyn, 1975). Before treatment was initiated and after therapy, ophthalmalogic examinations were performed and no eye changes were observed. One patient had taken 60 gm/day of DMSO for twenty months without any ocular ill-effects.

**Lens changes "species specific"**

During 1966, pharmaceutical companies gathered data on patients taking DMSO and no toxicity was observed. Merck collected 17,000 patient histories, Squibb, 3,000 patient reports, and Syntex, some 7,000 patient case reports. A conclusion was drawn that the lens changes were species specific and that primates were probably more resistant than other mammals.

**Vacaville tests validate safety**

Brobyn (1975) conducted a very extensive toxicological study during 1967-1968 at the State Prison in Vacaville, California, on prison inmates. DMSO was administered at three to thirty times the usual human dosage level for several months. During this time extensive diagnostic tests were conducted. These tests included eye examinations, blood and urine values, bone marrow studies, lung function, and heart studies. It was concluded that DMSO appears to be a safe drug for administration in humans. It was particularly determined that the eye changes occurring in certain mammalian species were not duplicatable in man under prolonged and high dosage treatment regimes.

Scherbel and colleagues (1967) reported the results of DMSO treatment on 61 scleraderma patients who had received a maximum dosage of 30 ml of 90 percent DMSO daily for periods up to 2¼ years. No eye toxicity was observed.

**Clinical side effects**

The most common and troublesome side effect of DMSO is the malodorous breath that occurs in the majority of the patients taking DMSO. This odor is generally described as an oyster- or garlic-like odor. Its intensity is generally directly related to the amount of DMSO that has been taken by a given patient. A portion of dimethyl sulfoxide is metabolized into dimethyl sulfide (DMS), which is exhaled by the patient and is responsible for this typical breath odor. Other than cessation of DMSO, no agent has yet been found to effectively counteract this odor.

**Malodorous breath**

An extensive research project was conducted in Germany (John and Laudahn, 1967) treating 4,180 patients with DMSO. Some of these patients were treated for over one year. Localized dermatitis occurred in 3.5 percent of the patients, a generalized dermatitis occurred in less than 0.1 percent. The intensity of the reaction generally was dependent on the area of application as well as the patient's type of skin. Patients with tender skin reacted more strongly. Furthermore, skin areas such as the neck, face, underarm, knee, and

**Localized dermatitis**

elbow joints were particularly sensitive to DMSO. It was necessary to use a lower concentration of the solution when treating these areas. In most patients with this localized skin reaction the treated area was reddened and clearly defined from nontreated skin. Another interesting observation was that the intensity of skin reaction varied from one application to another. Generally when a local skin reaction did occur, there was a tendency for it to decrease after each subsequent application. The affected skin would return to normal within two weeks after termination of DMSO application.

**Skin reactions explained**

The reason a local skin reaction occasionally occurs is that DMSO possesses a potent histamine-liberating property at the area of application (Jacob and Wood, 1971). It was found that this skin response would occur in the first week or two weeks of treatment and then disappear when the mast cell stores of histamine had been exhausted. None of the skin effects induced by topical DMSO are felt to be severe enough to warrant a contraindication to its use.

**Treatment of dermal irritation**

When a skin reaction does occur at the site of application, it is generally advisable to decrease the concentration of DMSO to a level where a reaction does not occur and then, after a short period of time, begin to increase the concentration once again. Increasing the concentration to 70 to 90 percent is usually required in order to receive optimal results for the condition being treated.

A frequent occurrence following topical application of DMSO is a slight burning or tingling sensation of the treated skin. This is followed generally by itching after the DMSO has begun to dry, usually within 15 to 30 minutes. These sensations are temporary and disappear within approximately a half an hour. With continued use of the drug these effects will be less intense (Steinberg, 1967). The use of a mild skin emollient such as *Aloe vera*, jojoba oil, or Vitamin E cream is helpful in alleviating these effects.

**Other side effects**

John and Laudahn further reported headaches and nausea in 1.6 percent of the patients treated. There were no reports nor clinical evidence of any changes in eyesight. No other effects were noted.

Brobyn (1975) in his extensive research project at the Vacaville State Prison on DMSO reported that the administration of 1.0gm/kg/day of DMSO over a long period of time was associated with some sedation, nausea, headaches, and dizziness. He did not observe any serious side effects. These findings are further collaborated by Jacob and Wood, as well as Steinberg, who also conducted extensive batteries of laboratory and diagnostic tests on patients receiving DMSO therapy.

**Toxicity of DMSO discussed**

DMSO is unquestionably one of the safest drugs available in the field of medicine when properly administered by a physician. No deaths have been reported by the use of the drug. However, for some unknown reason, the FDA has established a unique set of drug standards that are singular only to those compounds which they are intent upon keeping off the market.

**Drug standards inconsistent**

If the FDA were to apply the same drug standards to drugs now approved and in use as they have applied to DMSO, there would not be a single drug available in the United States today. The same standards that are imposed upon DMSO would also eliminate table salt, aspirin, alcoholic beverages, and cigarettes.

It is now estimated that over 6 million persons have used DMSO in one form or another as a therapeutic. Thus far no significant toxic side effects have been documented in humans that remotely justifies the suppressive action taken by the FDA.

# 5

# The Use of DMSO In The Treatment of Disease

**New Drug Approval granted**

In 1978, the FDA granted DMSO its first New Drug Approval (NDA) for use in man (FDA, 1980). This approval, although very specific and limited to application in bladder disorders, was a significant breakthrough for those struggling for the right to prescribe and use the drug.

**Interstitial cystitis**

This first FDA approval made available a 50 percent aqueous solution for the treatment of interstitial cystitis. Interstitial cystitis is a painful inflammation and irritation of the bladder of unknown origin, generally affecting females, yet also affecting some men. Symptoms include extreme frequency in voiding and pain over the bladder which is relieved by voiding.

The investigational use of DMSO in urology was initiated due to DMSO's noted efficacy in the treatment of various inflammatory conditions. The initial clinical report (Persky and Stewart, 1967) showed dramatic relief of pain was achieved when DMSO was instilled in the bladder. This study showed noted improvement in Peyronie's disease and epididymitis as well.

**Initial use of DMSO in urology**

Later clinical studies (Stewart and Shirley, 1976) showed satisfactory symptomatic relief in 75 percent of the patients treated with DMSO for interstitial cystitis and 80 percent of the patients were noted to be objectively improved. These patients received bladder instillations of 50ml of 50 percent DMSO every two weeks until maximum relief was obtained, then the intervals between treatments were decreased appropriately until treatment was discontinued.

It should be noted that in animal studies, dogs have received twice the volume per kilogram of body weight for twice the length of time at least 8 to 10 times more frequently than the dosage given to humans and there was no evidence of systemic or local toxicity.

Historically, the initial extensive clinical evaluation with DMSO in man concerned musculoskeletal disorders. These disorders received special attention due to various clinical trials sponsored by major pharmaceutical firms prior to the FDA ban on DMSO in 1965. These pharmaceutical firms were enthusiastic about the findings with DMSO and expended millions of dollars in support of the research up until 1965 (Herschler and Jacob, 1980).

**Muscle and skeleton disorders**

As will be reviewed in this section, excellent and often dramatic therapeutic results are seen in acute musculoskeletal inflammations and injuries. These exceptional results are achieved by a combination of various imposing properties DMSO possesses that include: anti-inflammatory activity with edema reduction, permeability of skin and other tissue, analgesic action to reduce pain, bacteriostatic and diuretic effects. These properties act in concert to bring about recovery in the majority of the patients with musculoskeletal and connective tissue disorders.

**Rheumatoid arthritis**

*Rheumatoid Arthritis:* Rheumatoid arthritis is a chronic disease characterized by inflammation of the joints of the upper and lower extremities. The disease often results in progressive destruction of those joints affected. As the disease progresses, the patient suffers from pain, inflammation, and a limitation of motion to the affected joint or joints. The cause of the disease is unknown.

A study was conducted in Germany on 177 rheumatoid arthritics (John and Laudahn, 1967). The patients were generally under treatment for six months. Routinely the patients' dosage of DMSO was 2 to 5ml of 90 percent DMSO applied two to four times daily over the affected area as well as the surrounding tissue. Seventy-four patients achieved complete remission of symptoms, 68 patients obtained partial remission, and only 35 received no benefit. The most dramatic response was in patients with minimal systemic involvement. The study indicated that long and continued periods of treatment were necessary.

**Continued treatment necessary**

Another clinical study was conducted in Japan (Matsumoto, 1967) involving 273 patients suffering with rheumatoid arthritis. The patients tested were limited to those rheumatoid arthritics with active involvement of the upper extremity joints. The study was only four weeks in length.

Prior to initiating treatment, during treatment, and following treatment, a complete series of diagnostic tests such as grip strength, joint circumference, range of motion, pain, and complete urine and blood tests were performed.

The patients were divided into three groups. One group was given a 90 percent DMSO solution, another group a 50 percent solution, and the third group was given a placebo substance. The patients applied their solutions to the affected areas of their bodies twice daily during the four weeks.

Significant results were observed with both of the groups treated with DMSO. DMSO relieved joint pain and increased grip strength and joint range of motion. DMSO proved most beneficial for patients whose illness had been of short duration and was at an early stage of development. The 90 percent solution was most effective.

Thirty-six rheumatoid arthritics were involved in a clinical study in New Jersey (Demos, et. al., 1967). A 90 percent DMSO solution was applied to the affected and surrounding tissue. The usual dosage was 0.1 to 0.2ml per kilogram body weight daily. Excellent to good results were observed in 50 percent of the patients tested.

**Recommended use of DMSO for arthritis**

The recommended area of application of DMSO for arthritis is the affected joint or joints and also a large area surrounding the joint. If a patient has arthritis of the hand, the entire hand and also half way up the forearm should receive application. In more severe cases, a series of intravenous infusions of DMSO may be implemented at the onset of treatment.

**Osteoarthritis**

*Osteoarthritis:* Osteoarthritis is a disease that affects joints and results in joint degeneration. The cause of the disease is unknown; however, aging, joint trauma, and obesity seem to create a tendency toward the disease. As the disease progresses, there is severe pain at the site of the affected joint. Muscle spasm and postural deformity may also occur.

**1641 patients studied**

The largest single clinical study of the effectiveness of DMSO in osteoarthritis was conducted in Germany (John and Laudahn, 1967) involving 1641 patients. The course of their treatment ranged from two to six months. Approximately 2 to 5ml of a 90 percent DMSO solution was applied to the affected and surrounding areas two to four times daily the first week, then reduced to twice daily until remission of symptoms occurred. Complete remission was obtained in

851 patients, partial recovery in 553 patients, and only 237 received no benefit from the use of DMSO.

A further report (Steinberg, 1967) describes findings with an additional 152 osteoarthritis patients. A 90 percent solution was applied to the affected joints and surrounding areas four times daily.

Patients noticed a significant decrease in pain within minutes of application, and the effect usually lasted four to six hours. A remarkable 84 percent showed significant results as evidenced by decreased swelling, pain relief, and increased mobility of the affected area.

**Recommended use of DMSO for osteoarthritis**

Because of the chronic nature of the disease, topical therapy must be maintained for months. When DMSO is used topically in osteoarthritis, it is imperative to also include the surrounding six-inch area as well as the affected joint for optimal results. In severe cases, a series of intravenous infusions of DMSO over a one-to-two week period at the onset of treatment is often the treatment of choice. In addition, a balanced nutritional and herbal supplement may be required. In severe cases of osteoarthritis the treatment may be further supplemented with the use of chelation therapy. See Halstead (1979, 1980) for further details on chelation therapy.

**Gouty arthritis**

*Gouty Arthritis:* Gouty arthritis is an acute disease of the joints of the extremities which may progress to become chronic and deforming. It is a disease that generally affects adult males. The disease is caused by a nutritional and metabolic disorder.

In a study conducted on 19 patients with gouty arthritis (John and Laudahn, 1967) receiving topical treatment with a 90 percent DMSO solution, 16 patients obtained complete remission of symptoms and three achieved partial remissions. There were no failures.

A further report (Blumenthal and Fuchs, 1967) on five patients receiving a 90 percent solution describes finding two patients with excellent results, two patients with good results, and one failure to respond to treatment.

**Recommended use of DMSO for gouty arthritis**

The general dosage in the treatment of gouty arthritis is 5ml of a 90 percent DMSO solution applied to the affected area and to the surrounding area two to four times daily until symptoms subside.

**Bursitis**

*Bursitis:* Bursitis is an inflamation of the bursa that surrounds the joint. The disease is characterized by pain, tenderness, swelling, and a limitation of motion to the involved joint. Bursitis may be caused by gouty infection, rheumatoid arthritis, or trauma.

An early report of clinical findings concerned a study of seven patients with acute bursitis (Rosenbaum and Jacob, 1964). Therapy involved topical application of 6 to 8ml of 90 percent DMSO solution to the affected area. Within 20 minutes all seven patients experienced pain relief and improved range of motion of the affected joint.

**Remarkable effects with bursitis**

A subsequent study was conducted on 1075 bursitis patients receiving DMSO treatment (John and Laudahn, 1967). Treatment consisted of approximately 5ml of 90 percent DMSO solution applied to the affected area two to four times daily. There were 293 patients suffering from acute bursitis. Complete remission was obtained by 136 patients, 121 patients obtained partial remission, and 36 patients showed no response to treatment. Of the 782 patients suffering from chronic bursitis, 345 received complete remission, 321 patients obtained partial remission, and 116 showed no improvement following three months of DMSO therapy.

Further proof of the effectiveness of DMSO treatment in bursitis was reported in a clinical study involving 141 patients (Demos, et. al., 1967). A 90 percent solution was applied liberally to affected areas and surrounding tissues. Good to excellent response was observed in 73 percent of the patients with acute bursitis and 57 percent in chronic bursitis.

In the experience of Parsons, et. al. (1967), relief of pain and an increase in range of motion was achieved in 90 percent of the patients suffering from chronic frozen shoulder.

**Tendonitis and peritendonitis**

*Tendonitis and Peritendonitis:* Tendonitis and peritendonitis are characterized by inflammation of the tendons and their surrounding area and can occur in various areas of the body; however, the most common occurrence is at the shoulder, wrist, elbow, ankle, and knee. It may be due to excess use of the area or to a single or repeated injury. Symptoms of the disease are local pain and inflammation.

A report of a study on 50 patients (Steinberg, 1967) showed that a remarkable 94 percent of the patients received most favorable results. The treatment given was 90 percent DMSO solution applied liberally to the area every four hours initially, then decreased for the duration of the treatment. The response to the DMSO was rapid, generally within ten to fifteen minutes following application.

**Chronic back disorders**

*Back Pain and Disc Disorders:* There can be various causes for acute or chronic back disorders. There could be a local mechanical defect or injury present, a structural inadequacy, an intervertebral disc abnormality or disease, or an abnormality elsewhere in the body contributing to the disorder.

The ability of DMSO to be effective in disorders of the back is largely determined by the cause of the disorder. DMSO does have the ability to decrease pain and inflammation; however, if there is a mechanical or structural cause underlying the pain, its effects will only be transitory at best.

A study was conducted in Washington, D.C., on 17 patients with chronic back pain (Blumenthal and Fuchs, 1967) that were treated with a topical application of 90 percent DMSO several times daily over a period of two days to eight months. Four patients obtained excellent results, nine received good results, and four reported no improvement.

**Discogenic disease**

Another clinical study was conducted on 18 patients with discogenic disease (Steinberg, 1967). These patients were treated with applications of 90 percent DMSO every four to six hours. The patients with recent injury or acute illness responded more quickly and readily than the patients with chronic back disorders. The overall positive response in both groups was 50 percent. Of those that did achieve excellent results, relapses were uncommon.

**Sprains, strains, whiplash and athletic injuries**

*Sprains, Strains, Whiplash and Athletic Injuries:* Some of the most striking and gratifying results in DMSO therapy have been obtained in patients suffering with tissue injury because of DMSO's ability to decrease inflammation, improve circulation to the injured area, and to promote pain relief. Often when treating patients with these injuries, the use of splints, elastic bandages, and adhesive taping can be discarded. Frequently within one to two hours of treatment there is almost complete relief of pain and tenderness. The incapacity of the patient being treated can be substantially lessened and the time loss from work can be greatly reduced in patients receiving DMSO.

A clinical study on 223 patients with sprain injuries and 145 strain injury patients was conducted (Demos, et.al., 1967) using topically applied 90 percent DMSO liberally to the involved area several times daily. Excellent results were obtained in 83 percent of the patients with sprain injuries and 67 percent in strain injury patients.

In Germany another study was conducted on 479 patients with sprains, strains, and tissue contusions (John and Laudahn, 1967). The patients received 2 to 5ml topical

90 percent DMSO two to four times daily immediately following injury and for the first week; then the dosage was reduced to once or twice daily until remission of symptoms occurred. Complete remission of symptoms was achieved in 325 patients, partial remission in 95, and only 59 patients showed no response to DMSO treatment.

A study conducted in Pennsylvania (Steinberg, 1967) involved 53 acute injury patients. This group consisted of not only sprain and strain patients, but also whiplash and back injury as well as other acute tissue injury. The patients were given a topical 90 percent DMSO solution every four to six hours initially. Application was repeated as often as necessary to relieve pain and assure mobility thereafter. Generally, the patients treated noticed evidence of pain relief within 20 minutes which lasted an average of four hours. A favorable response, evidenced by motion restoration and pain relief, was achieved in 81 percent of the patients treated.

**Rapid pain relief obtained**

Blumenthal and Fuchs (1967) reported on 29 patients with acute musculoskeletal injuries who received topical 90 percent DMSO therapy for only two to eight days. Excellent results were obtained in 12 patients, good results in 11 patients, and 6 patients obtained poor results.

Luth (Jacob and Wood, 1967), of Germany, treated over 400 patients with DMSO who had received athletic injuries and found DMSO to be the drug of choice in their treatment. Also, Dr. Paul, the team physician for the Toronto Mapleleafs baseball team made a comparative study of DMSO with his athletes. He found that time lost due to injury in the year DMSO was used was 28 days, whereas the previous year's loss was 42 days. These results are significant because professional athletes have strong motivation to return to work as soon as possible. Paul concluded that DMSO was the drug of choice in treating athletic injuries.

**Study conducted with professional athletes**

Fractures

*Fractures:* It has been found that DMSO is a useful adjunct in the treatment of fractures where inflammation and/or persistent pain are present.

A clinical report on 147 bone fracture patients (John and Laudahn, 1967) in which a 90 percent DMSO solution was applied to the affected area several times daily showed 88 patients received excellent results, 39 good results, and 20 failed to achieve benefit from therapy.

The use of DMSO in patients with one fracture is further supported by Blumenthal and Fuchs (1967). Seven patients with hip, rib, and toe fractures were treated with 90 percent DMSO over the fractured areas. All patients were benefited, three obtained good results, four received excellent results. DMSO kept the patients quite comfortable without the use of pain medication. Two other patients received similar treatment with DMSO (Steinberg, 1967) for rib fractures and hip fractures, and both obtained excellent results.

Osteomyelitis

*Osteomyelitis:* Osteomyelitis is a serious infection of the bone marrow. It also may spread to surrounding tissue and skin surfaces and form abcesses if treatment and response to treatment is not achieved promptly. Vigorous antibiotic treatment is the therapy of choice.

A case history of a patient with osteomyelitis was presented at a symposium on DMSO at the New York Academy of Sciences (Sanders, 1967). The patient was a 48-year-old male who had contracted osteomyelitis 30 years previously. The initial diagnosis had been made at Massachusetts General Hospital and confirmed at other centers during the long course of the disease. Various antibiotic compounds had been used without affecting the rampant bacteria in the bone of his leg. Finally, amputation became the only apparent solution that could save his life. However, there was no guarantee that even this drastic measure would be effective in controlling the disease process.

Amputation avoided

The patient had strenuously and consistently insisted he would not submit to leg amputation. Therefore, as a last recourse and with no prior knowledge of DMSO's effectiveness in osteomyelitis, DMSO therapy was initiated. Treatment consisted of topical irrigations of the purulent leg wound over a six-month period. The patient received 46 irrigations of approximately 3oz of DMSO per irrigation. Initially a 50 percent DMSO, 10 percent glycerine, and 40 percent water solution was administered. Then the dosage was increased to 90 percent DMSO and 10 percent glycerine.

Finally, after an illness of over 30 years and after only six months of DMSO therapy, there was a complete cessation of the infection. The patient's recovery was most remarkable.

Unfortunately, no other clinical studies are available on this disease.

**Dupuytren's contracture**

*Dupuytren's Contracture:* This disorder is characterized by a thickening, shortening, and fibrosis of the muscles of the hands or feet causing deformity of the fingers or toes.

At the DMSO Symposium in Vienna, Wodniansky reported treating 22 patients suffering from Dupuytren's contracture with topical DMSO. Eleven patients noted improvement and he determined DMSO treatment was of particular value in the early stages of the disease (Jacob and Wood, 1967).

A further report (Rosenbaum, et. al., 1965) on three patients treated with 30ml topical DMSO applied daily showed that all three obtained improvement within three months. There was increased range of finger motion as well as a reduction of the plaque size of the affected extremity following DMSO therapy.

**Scleroderma**

*Scleroderma:* Scleroderma is a disorder of unknown cause in which there is a sclerosis or calcifying of connective tissue. It is a disease with no known cure.

The course of scleroderma is extremely variable and unpredictable. It can move slowly or swiftly through the patient. The general early manifestation of the disease is a sclerosis or tightening of the skin in the arms or legs. The disease progresses to form ulcerations of the fingertips, ankles, or elbows. As circulation is choked off, gangrene of the extremities may set in.

**Scleroderma progression**

As scleroderma progresses it may cause a thickening and hardening of the connective tissues of various organs, the heart or lungs, as well as other vital organs. Joint movement becomes painful and muscle atrophy occurs, greatly limiting any movement of the patient.

The use of DMSO in scleroderma has been studied by various investigators since Scherbel, et. al. (1965) published a report on the treatment of ten patients with DMSO. A further report (Scherbel, et. al., 1967) gives an account of findings with 42 scleroderma cases. The improvements noted included a softening of the skin, increased grip strength and finger movement, and the disappearance of collagen bundles. Furthermore, the skin ulcers would generally heal in one to six weeks following initiation of treatment. Of these 42 patients, 26 showed good to excellent improvement and 16 showed fair to poor response.

Further clinical studies cited by Herschler and Jacob (1980) were conducted in the Soviet Union (Sergayev and Zakiev, 1967) using 30 to 90 percent DMSO on a large group of scleroderma patients over a six to thirty month period of time. Their clinical findings closely matched those of Scherbel.

**Disease undergoing positive change**

It should be emphasized that the results seen in these scleroderma patients treated with DMSO have not been observed with any other presently employed therapy. This is the first evidence that the disease process is undergoing a positive change. Chelation therapy, when administered with DMSO, has been found to enhance the clinical improvement of scleroderma patients.

**Recommended use**

The DMSO dosage for the scleroderma patient is generally between 50gm to 75gm daily. Most patients do not tolerate the same dose concentration on all parts of the body. Some areas, such as the face, neck, and underarms, are more sensitive than other parts of the body and the DMSO concentrate must be lowered to possibly 60 percent or the patient's tolerance level. Other areas, such as the back, legs, and arms, may tolerate strengths up to 95 percent.

Generally, at the beginning of treatment, DMSO is applied topically to the entire body in concentrations of 60 to 90 percent, as tolerated. The DMSO is allowed to penetrate the skin until it is absorbed, usually about twenty to thirty minutes. After two or three weeks the administration should be restricted to the hands, forearms, and feet, and occasionally the face. This is repeated three times daily for approximately three months, then reduced to twice daily until softening of the skin occurs.

When a patient shows poor response to topical DMSO application, immersion of the hands, wrists, or feet in 50 percent DMSO will often give beneficial results.

**Neurologic disorders**

*Central Nervous System Trauma:* Spinal cord, head injuries, and strokes are complex neurologic problems confronting medicine today. Over the years conventional treatment has not been very effective.

**Central nervous system trauma**

The pathologic process involved in brain and spinal cord injuries is generally a complex combination of nerve injury involving a lack of oxygen, diminished blood flow, and involving edema. The wide range of action DMSO possesses has been found to be useful in treating many of these neurological conditions.

There are three unique properties of DMSO that make it a highly desirable agent in treating spinal cord and head injuries. It provides protection of cells from mechanical damage (Ashwood-Smith, 1967), strong diuresis (Formanek, et. al., 1966), and reduction of tissue edema (Formanek and Kovacs, 1966; Gorog and Kovacs, 1968).

Dr. Jack de la Torre, et. al. (1975) at the University of Chicago School of Medicine conducted three significant studies in neurological trauma:

**Middle cerebral artery occlusion**

Middle Cerebral Artery Occlusion: Massive strokes were induced in monkeys by exposing a middle cerebral artery and closing it with a clip for four hours. After the removal of the clip, controlled experiments were begun on various groups of the animals.

The animals that showed the most remarkable recovery with little or no paralysis was the group given DMSO or DMSO in combination with hyperbaric oxygen therapy. Animals in the control group or those treated by other modalities had a significantly lower survival rate as well as a higher degree of subsequent muscle weakness and paralysis.

**Spinal cord injury**

Spinal Cord Injury: A study was conducted on dogs following controlled injury of their spinal cords. Motor recovery was accelerated by DMSO given immediately after spinal cord compression. Dogs treated with hyperbaric oxygen also experienced more rapid motor recovery. The study showed a significant reversal of paralysis in the DMSO group that was remarkable. The critical factors were the dosage and time of treatment after injury.

**Head injury**

Head Injury: Controlled brain compression injuries were inflicted on monkeys in an experiment to simulate an extradural hematoma as frequently occurs in severe head injuries. There were significant observations that were remarkable. DMSO reduced intracranial pressure to normal levels and improved blood flow to the brain. It also protected against neurologic deficits such as paralysis. The mortality rate on the control group was 100 percent, whereas in the group treated with DMSO it was only 7 percent.

More recently (de la Torre, 1977), studies have been conducted using DMSO on patients with recent brain and spinal cord injury. Most of the permanent neurological damage in these patients is caused by a reduction of blood flow to the brain which induces an inadequate supply of nutrients as well as oxygen to delicate brain tissue. Through a combination of dehydration and hyperosmosis (increased fluid diffusion across body membranes) it relieves damaging pressure and swelling that may accompany spinal cord and head trauma. This feat is accomplished by DMSO's unique ability to cross both the dermal and blood-brain barriers. DMSO enters the tissue, picks up water rapidly, then is excreted from the system, relieving excess pressure.

**Blood-brain barrier penetrated**

This ability to penetrate dermal and blood-brain barriers without damaging cells unquestionably places DMSO in a class by itself. Equally unique in this sense is its ability to protect cells from mechanical damage.

**Reversal of paralysis**

Patients with spinal cord injury, stroke, or head injury must initiate DMSO treatment within no more than four hours of onset of injury or the pathological consequences may be irreversible. Patients who have initiated treatment within this critical time framework have had remarkable reversal of paralysis as well as return of consciousness following stroke or head trauma. It is during this same period of time that hyperbaric oxygen therapy is most effective, but it is also not generally used by conventional medicine, much to the detriment of the patient.

Hopefully, in the not too distant future, DMSO will be available in emergency rooms, ambulances, and paramedical units, and emergency medical personnel will be properly educated and trained so many of these tragically crippling neurological disorders can be reversed before damage becomes permanent.

**Headache**

*Headache:* There are many types of headaches, just as there are many causes or psychological reasons for headaches to occur. In Washington, D.C., a study was conducted on 154 patients with various types of headaches, neuralgia, and neck pain (Blumenthal and Fuchs, 1967). The patients were treated with a 90 percent DMSO solution applied topically to the painful area, whether it was the face, scalp, or neck region. Approximately 3 to 10ml of DMSO was used at each application and was repeated twice daily for chronic conditions and in more severe headaches it was repeated up to every three hours.

Excellent results were obtained in 35 patients, 60 patients received good results, and 59 patients obtained no noted relief. Most of the vascular and migrane headaches, and face pain, generally tended to respond poorly to DMSO. Good response was obtained by patients with temporal arthritis. When headaches were due to muscle spasm, cervical arthritis, or disc disorders, the results obtained by the patients were much more satisfactory. When headaches were due to a recent injury or disease such as sinusitis, the results obtained were generally excellent.

A further report on a study of ten patients with vascular headaches indicated a much more dramatic response was obtained by the patients that were treated with DMSO for vascular headaches (Ogden, 1967). A 90 percent DMSO solution was again used and applied directly to the painful area.

The results of this study were a remarkable 100 percent remission for all patients treated with DMSO. Furthermore, it was apparent that the quicker the DMSO was applied after the onset of the headache, the more rapid the pain relief was obtained.

**Post-amputation pain**

*Post-Amputation Pain:* Eight patients suffering from post-amputation phantom pain were treated with 30ml of 90 to 100 percent DMSO (Stewart and Jacob, 1965). The strength of the DMSO was diluted with water or glycerine to avert skin reaction, then applied in two doses daily. In six of the eight patients the initial treatment relieved the phantom pain for up to four hours. As treatment continued, there was progressively longer periods of pain relief and the patients were able to discontinue analgesic and sedative medication they had taken prior to this time. All patients were able to discontinue therapy within three months.

**Neuritis**

*Neuritis:* Local neuritis is a disease that generally involves a single nerve. It is usually caused by trauma, an inflammation, chilling, or loss of blood supply.

A study was conducted on 88 patients with acute neuritis (Steinberg, 1967). They were treated with 90 percent DMSO applied to the affected area every four to six hours. Pain relief occurred within five to ten minutes and generally lasted four to six hours. All the patients treated responded favorably.

**Tic Douloureux**

*Tic Douloureux:* Tic douloureux, also known as trigeminal neuralgia, is a disorder in which there are brief attacks of severe pain in one or more branches of the facial trigeminal nerve.

A study was conducted on 35 tic douloureux patients (Jacob, 1965) that were treated with 60ml of 50 percent DMSO which was applied to the face twice daily. When the pain originated in the nasal area, no more than 2ml of DMSO was applied to the mucous area daily. Of the 35 patients treated, 26 achieved significant improvement. Initially, pain relief lasted two to three hours after DMSO treatment. As treatment progressed, the periods of relief increased. Generally, significant pain relief was obtained within three to four days.

**Multiple Sclerosis**

*Multiple Sclerosis:* The cause of this disease is unknown. There is a slow breaking down of the brain and spinal cord lining which causes interruption of neurologic functions and spasticity. While it has been reported that DMSO is beneficial in the treatment of multiple sclerosis, this does not appear to be the response of the average patient. Most obtained no positive benefit.

**Case history**

A multiple sclerosis patient undergoing treatment in Oregon did receive positive benefit (McGrady, 1973). She was paralyzed and also had some kidney damage prior to her beginning DMSO therapy under Dr. Jacob. Two ounces of DMSO was applied topically to her body daily in addition to her taking DMSO orally in orange or tomato juice.

Her condition began to improve dramatically. Within one week, her kidney disorder began to improve. Then, in a matter of weeks, she could walk again. Six years after her initial DMSO treatments she is still able to walk, however manifestations of multiple sclerosis are still present.

A study reported on by Herschler and Jacob (1970) involved six multiple sclerosis patients who also found significant improvements with this disease following DMSO therapy. The patients were given daily topical applications of 30 to 60ml DMSO for a course of two weeks. Following the two-week treatment, all patients manifested definite improvement including disappearance of numbness, improved bladder control, relief of double vision, and increased clarity of speech. Furthermore, areas of muscle spasm which were swabbed with 5 to 15ml of DMSO obtained definite relaxation of the affected muscle within thirty minutes of application.

In the treatment of multiple sclerosis at the Halstead Preventive Medical Clinic, there is clinical evidence that multiple sclerosis patients attain further improvements when DMSO is combined with hyperbaric oxygen therapy and Oil of Evening Primrose, which contains linoleic acid.

**Neoplastic disease**

Cancer is one of the leading causes of death in the United States today. Billions of dollars and an enormous manpower research effort has been expended in search of a cure for this dreaded disease. Dozens of clinical trials have been conducted using DMSO alone or in combination with other agents to combat malignant diseases. Two very positive findings have resulted from animal experiments. A study conducted in Austria on mice revealed that DMSO increased the production of interferon two to sixteen fold when the mice were infected with viruses (Kunze, 1975). Interferon is a class of small proteins produced by cells of the body that inhibit viruses and are believed to be useful against cancer.

Another study conducted in New York on rabbits (Bartfield and Goldstein, 1975) revealed that DMSO potentiated cell-mediated immunity, that is, it caused stimulation of the immune system of the body thus giving a boost to the body to heal itself when subjected to malignancy or infection.

**Leukemia**

*Leukemia:* Leukemia is a generalized neoplastic disorder of blood-forming tissues with a primary effect on leukocyte or white blood cell formation and production. As in the other types of cancer, the cause is unknown, however, certain environmental factors may play a key role in its evolution. The course of the disease varies not only with the type of leukemia present, but also with each individual and therapy employed.

In a laboratory study conducted in Florida it was found that organisms isolated from tumor and leukemia patients stopped growing when exposed to a 25 percent DMSO solution (Seibert, et. al., 1967). Furthermore, there was no damage or change noted in normal cell growth patterns. Another study (Dennis and Wilson, 1975) found that DMSO proved preferentially toxic to leukemia cells as compared to its effect on normal white blood cells. This research was further substantiated by Schrek, et. al., (1967) which showed

DMSO proved to be less toxic to white blood cells of non-leukemia patients.

Several studies have also shown that DMSO actually has the ability to enduce erythroleukemic differentiation, or in other words, revert leukemia cells back to a normal type of cell (Marks and Rifkind, 1978; Marks, et. al., 1979).

**Malignant tumors**

*Malignant Tumors:* A very significant finding in the use of DMSO is that it affects the growth pattern of tumor cells when in culture, inducing drastic change from the bizarre growth of tumor cells to a growth pattern that closely resembles the growth of normal cells (Borenfreund, et. al., 1975). This effect was reversible when the tumor cells were withdrawn from DMSO. It appeared that DMSO affected cell membrane components leading to structural changes on the cell surface.

Another laboratory study on rats (Fletcher and Dennis, 1967) revealed that DMSO may actually suppress the appearance of tumors. After the 18-month study period, the rats receiving DMSO had fewer tumors and weighed more than the control group. However, another study (Armstrong and Cohn, 1967) on rabbits where DMSO was instilled in their abdomens and observation of tumor growth was made, there was indication that DMSO alone did not have any effect on tumor growth.

**Drug potentiating abilities**

In various studies, DMSO has been used in combination with other agents where it enhances their effects by assisting not only with more adequate tissue penetration, but also its potentiation effect on many concurrently administered drugs.

A study was conducted on female patients with pre-cancerous and cancerous growths in cervical carcinoma (Ayre and LeGuerrier, 1967). Pure DMSO applications showed no changes in the cervix of the patients tested, however, when a 90 percent DMSO and .01 percent decadron (a steroid) was applied to the lesions, regression of this disease appeared within two to three weeks.

A research project was designed by Warren, et. al., (1975) to evaluate the effectiveness of combining DMSO with various anticancer drugs. They found that when large doses of DMSO were combined with Cytoxan, a highly toxic chemotherapy agent closely akin to nitrogen mustard, and given to cancerous rats, the rats died quite rapidly. DMSO alone had no ill effects. Therefore, the DMSO was given at low concentrations, one and two percent, along with a low dose of the chemotherapy drug. This increased the therapeutic effect and antitumor action of the drug which also lowered the toxic threshold. This is most significant in that the highly toxic and adverse effects which chemotherapy agents have on the immune system and body as a whole may be drastically reduced by their administration in low doses in combination with DMSO.

**Tested with anti-cancer drugs**

In Chile, a study was conducted on 65 cancer patients using DMSO, Cytoxan, and amino acids (Cornejo and Lagos, 1975). The patients received extensive diagnostic tests prior to and during this chemotherapy trial. Many of the patients had received conventional cancer therapy prior to this time that proved fruitless.

The patients were given low doses of the chemotherapy agent combined with DMSO and amino acids every day or every other day until a specified minimum dosage had been administered. The tolerance of the chemotherapy by the patients was remarkable. White blood cell suppression or malformation was scarce or absent and there was a marked relief of pain observed by the patients.

**Tolerance to chemotherapy improved**

Summary of the results are as follows: of eight Hodgkin's disease patients, seven had good response and remission; of ten lymphosarcoma patients, all obtained remission; of three bone sarcoma patients, all received remissions; one patient who was treated for Ewing's tumor also obtained remission. There were 26 patients that were treated for breast cancer, all of whom had metastases. Remission was obtained in 23 patients and three showed no improvement.

**Various cancers affected by DMSO**

**DMSO and Laetrile**

DMSO has been used by many clinicians in combination with amygdalin (Laetrile) and metabolic cancer therapy. It assists in the dispersement and assimilation of amygdalin and other nutrients given to the cancer patient as well as plays an important role in the enhancement of interferon production and immune stimulation.

**Cardiovascular disorders**

*Ischemia of the Heart* (Coronary Artery Disease): There are many heart problems that are associated with ischermia which is caused by a lack of or decreased supply of oxygen to the heart muscle due to coronary artery disease.

An animal study was conducted in Texas treating the ischemic heart with DMSO and with DMSO combined with hydrogen peroxide (Finney, et. al., 1967). While it was noted that a dilute hydrogen peroxide can be used as an oxygen source by the heart, the addition of DMSO resulted in maintenance of a functioning heart. DMSO aided oxygen diffusion throughout the heart muscle thus protecting against oxygen loss.

**Coronary artery disease**

Further clinical trials were conducted on whole hearts perfused with DMSO (Herschler and Jacob, 1980). The functional effects on the heart were a concentration dependent decrease in heartbeat and a positive effect on heart contractability. It is suggested that DMSO may relieve transient heart ischermia thus being useful as a heart stimulant.

**Chronic venous insufficiency**

*Chronic Venous Insufficiency:* Vascular disorders of the peripheral circulation may be caused by disease in the peripheral arterial system, a disturbance in the nervous system, or by an organic vascular disease such as atherosclerosis. After the flow of blood to an area has been restricted for some time, adaptive changes may occur in the extremity affected.

A study was conducted in Switzerland on 55 patients with chronic venous insufficiency (Widmer, Glaus, and Raps, 1972). One half of these patients were treated with a placebo and half were given a DMSO solution combined with anti-inflammatory agents. After a two-week trial, the group treated with the DMSO solution obtained clearly superior results over the placebo group.

**Other venous disorders**

Another study in Switzerland (Kappert, 1975) treating 59 patients with venous disorders of the extremities with DMSO combined with anti-inflammatory agents showed significant benefit was obtained by the patients treated. Excellent results were obtained by 35 patients, fair response obtained by 12 patients, and 12 patients noticed no significant improvement.

**Thrombophlebitis and phlebitis**

*Thrombophlebitis and Phlebitis:* These disorders are caused by an inflammation of the vein wall in which there might be a blood clot present. These disorders are generally the result of trauma, prolonged inactivity, a blood coagulation disorder, or bacterial infection. Superficial thrombophlebitis and phlebitis are manifested by a reddened, heated, and painful tract of skin that is swollen and sensitive to touch.

DMSO was used experimentally in rats in the treatment of induced thrombophlebitis (Gorog and Kovacs, 1975). It was found that DMSO was effective against blood clot formation, inflammation, and promoted restoration of blood flow to the diseased area.

A double-blind clinical study was conducted in Switzerland on patients with superficial thrombophlebitis (Nachbar, 1972). A DMSO preparation was used that also contained inflammation-inhibiting drugs prednisone and diphenyl butazone. This solution was used by 23 patients and was applied by spray to the entire inflammed skin area and allowed to dry. The application was repeated three times daily for five days.

The control group consisted of 24 thrombophlebitis patients and they were also given a placebo spray to apply in the identical manner the DMSO group used their spray.

Following the five-day trial, all patients were evaluated. Criteria used were skin temperature of affected area as well as beneath the skin, degree of skin redness, the amount of swelling present, and patients' subjective responses concerning pain and sensitivity to pressure. Of the 23 patients treated with the DMSO preparation, 16 received excellent results and 7 obtained no significant benefit. In the control group of 24 patients, 10 noticed relief and 14 patients observed no improvement.

A similar study was also conducted in Switzerland (Kappert, 1975) on 48 phlebitis patients using approximately the same DMSO solution with added anti-inflammatory agents. Excellent results were obtained by 30 patients, fair response by 6 patients, and 12 received no noticeable benefit.

An investigation in Canada (Paul, 1967) employed a 70 percent DMSO solution alone in treating four patients with thrombophlebitis. Three patients suffering from acute thrombophlebitis obtained excellent results, one patient with chronic thrombitis received good results.

**Varicose veins**

*Varicose Veins:* Varicose veins are abnormally dilated and lengthened superficial veins that occur because the valves in the veins become incompetent and are unable to pump the blood out of the legs rapidly enough to prevent the high pressure in the affected vein or veins. Certain forces such as prolonged standing or pregnancy tend to augment the venous pressure in the lower extremities.

A study was conducted in Canada (Paul, 1967) on 22 patients with varicose veins and associated cramping disorders. A 70 percent solution was liberally applied to the varicosity affected limbs. The patients, aged 22 to 72, were treated for a minimum of eight weeks. Twenty-one of the 22 patients treated obtained either good or excellent results manifested by cramping reduction or disappearance, diminished edema, and actual fading of the "spiders" that often accompany varicosities.

Gangrene

*Gangrene:* Gangrene is a disease that occurs because of decreased blood supply which causes a lack of oxygen delivery to the involved tissue. The primary reason DMSO is a treatment of choice in gangrene patients is that DMSO increases the blood flow to the affected area due to its vasodilatory properties, thus limiting the spread of the disease (Jacob, 1979).

In the treatment of gangrene at the Halstead Preventive Medical Clinic, topical DMSO in concentrations of 70 to 80 percent is applied liberally to the healthy tissue adjacent to the gangrenous area and not to the diseased area. This treatment is augmented by hyperbaric oxygen therapy and chelation therapy (see Halstead, 1979, 1980). Encouraging results have been obtained combining these modalities in the treatment of early gangrene.

Respiratory disorders

*Chronic Respiratory Insufficiency:* This disease is a condition in which gases such as oxygen in the arterial blood stream cannot be maintained within the normal limits necessary for optimum health.

Chronic respiratory insufficiency

A study was conducted in Chile (Marin, 1975) on 43 patients with chronic respiratory insufficiency. These patients were divided into two groups, one group to be given aminophylline, a drug routinely used in disorders of this type, and the other group to be given a DMSO preparation. Prior to initiation of the treatments, the patients underwent extensive diagnostic testing which was repeated at the conclusion of the study.

Both groups of patients received daily intramuscular injections of their respective medications for twenty consecutive days. Every three days during this period of time blood was taken and arterial blood measurements were made.

The results of the study indicated the group given

DMSO received significant benefit, both in symptomatic relief and in improvement in their arterial blood values.

**Bronchiolitis and acute bronchitis**

*Bronchiolitis and Acute Bronchitis:* These disorders are characterized by an inflammatory obstruction of the respiratory tract, generally starting with an acute respiratory infection and progressive respiratory difficulties and coughing.

In Chile (Zuniga, et. al., 1975) a study was conducted on 60 infants with bronchiolitis and acute respiratory obstruction. One half of the infants were controls and were treated with antibiotics, oxygen, and steam tent treatment only. The DMSO group was given the same treatment, but also an aerosol spray was administered. This spray contained an anti-inflammatory drug, a bacteriostatic drug, and DMSO. The DMSO was used because of its penetrating and drug-potentiation ability. A dose of 2ml of the DMSO spray was applied to the back of the throat of the infants and repeated 1 to 4 times as the child's condition indicated.

The results of this study showed that approximately thirty minutes after the initial DMSO treatment, 80 percent of the infants obtained sensorial and coughing improvement and 75 percent of the infants had improved breathing ability and decreased respiratory rate. Furthermore, there was a deferred effect in the DMSO group in that the DMSO spray reduced the necessity to use a steam tent on the patients. The spray had a tendency to decrease the inflammatory process and to reduce the viscosity (stickiness) of the respiratory secretions so they could be more readily coughed up by the infants.

**Asthma**

*Asthma:* Another investigation was conducted in Chile (Bernath, et. al., 1980). This study was carried out on 153 patients with asthma, a disease where there is an obstruction of air flow to the lungs. The patients had suffered with asthma for from one to six years. Prior to treatment and following the study the patients were given extensive diagnostic tests. The course of therapy consisted of DMSO combined with a bronchodilator, an antihistamine, and an anti-inflammatory steroid that was given to the patients daily by intramuscular injection over a 15 to 20 day period. Excellent results were obtained in 24 percent of the patients, good results were obtained in 60 percent, and 15 percent noticed no change.

**Skin disorders and infectious disease**

*Psoriasis:* Psoriasis is a disease of the skin characterized by a sharply demarcated elevation of the skin that is slightly scaly. It is generally a chronic condition with frequent relapses.

**Psoriasis**

In Georgia, a study was conducted on psoriasis patients using DMSO alone as therapy (Engel, 1967). The patients showed improvement during the initial seven to ten days of treatment, then the results were disasterous. All of the patients became worse. They did notice, however, that the itching was relieved by the DMSO. Research is continuing using a steroid-DMSO combination for psoriasis treatment and the results appear more promising.

A study conducted in the Lanchow General Hospital in China was reported in the *Chinese Medical Journal* in 1975 (Ching-jung and Hsi-shan, 1975). Thirty-three patients with acute psoriasis were given an extract of camptotheca nuts combined with DMSO. After a few weeks of treatment, 21 patients had received excellent results; all eruptions had disappeared. The other 12 patients were greatly improved.

**Chronic skin ulcers**

*Chronic Skin Ulcers and Infected Wounds:* An extensive study was done in Chile on patients with chronic skin ulcers (Miranda-Tirado, 1975). A total of 1,371 patients received DMSO for skin ulcers due to various causes such as infected ulcerations, chronic diabetic ulcers, and second- or third-degree burns of the extremities.

DMSO spray was used as the exclusive therapy; no other medication was employed. Generally, the DMSO was administered topically to the affected area three times weekly. Prior to application, the wound area was cleansed of exudate, dead tissue, and foreign material. They found that 95 percent of the 1,371 patients obtained excellent results with complete healing of the affected wound. After the first application of DMSO, the majority of the patients noticed immediate pain relief. One patient with chronic diabetic ulcers for the past 15 years received complete wound healing after 20 days of DMSO therapy.

One of the observations made in this study was that chronic chain smokers and alcoholics received favorable results; however, their wounds healed more slowly.

**Infected wounds**

A clinical trial was conducted in the Soviet Union on 54 patients with infected surgical wounds (Bayare, et. al., 1971). A 60 percent DMSO solution was used. The patients treated received a prompt reduction of swelling around the wound, obtained effective pain relief, and rapid recovery of the wound. It was found to have an anti-microbial effect on the wound infection as well.

Another study in the Soviet Union was conducted on 210 patients with inflammed purulent wounds (Dubinsky and Skager, 1975). These patients were treated with 40 percent DMSO combined with antibiotics. Positive results were seen in the patients treated. Pain and swelling were diminished, there was a cleansing of the wound and rapid healing of the tissues was noted. The work of Dubinsky and Skager was supported by Golamozov (1970) in his laboratory research conducted on infectious wounds in dogs.

**Gum infections**

*Gum Infections:* A study was conducted in Poland on 15 patients with paradontitis, an inflammation and bleeding of the gum tissue (Krzywicki and Rewerska, 1966). The patients were treated with a 40 percent DMSO solution. Excellent results were observed in all patients as noted by a cessation of gum bleeding and pain and by healing of the gum tissue.

Patients have also reported excellent results from the use of DMSO (80 percent solution) in the treatment of canker sores of the mucous membranes of the mouth.

**Herpes zoster**

*Herpes Zoster:* This particular type of herpes is better known to the layman as shingles. It is characterized by eruptions and pain that follow nerve pathways under the skin that is affected. The disease is caused by an acute viral infection of the central nervous system.

A study conducted by Sehtman (1975) on 7 patients with herpes zoster showed excellent results were obtained by all patients treated with DMSO.

**Herpes simplex**

*Herpes Simplex:* This type of herpes is commonly referred to as a fever blister or cold sore. It is characterized by a small cluster of inflammed vesicles that appear on the skin or mucus membranes. It is caused by a virus infection.

A study was conducted in Argentina using DMSO on 10 patients with herpes simplex (Sehtman, 1975). Four lesions were on the lip, two on the chest, and four on the penis. Spectacular success was obtained within 48 hours in all patients. They had received two applications per day. It is felt that it is important to initiate DMSO treatment as soon as the sore appears.

Another study was conducted on 7 patients with severe recurrent herpes simplex infections (Goldman and Kitzmiller, 1965). Treatment was initiated within two days following the initial manifestation of the disease. A preparation of 90 percent DMSO and 10 percent water was combined with a one percent solution of 5-iodo-2′-dioxyuride and applied sparingly to the affected area four times daily.

The patient treated within 12 hours after the onset of the redness developed no lesion, a first in a long history of recurrences for this patient. Another patient with a lesion of the eyebrow attained resolution within 48 hours. A patient with severe recurrent gluteal herpes simplex obtained prompt relief of pain with no recurrence during treatment.

A patient with hemorrhagic gluteal herpes simplex attained subsidence of lesions within 48 hours. In all the other patients, subsidence of lesions was achieved in 48 hours, along with scaling and drying of the affected area.

**Burns**

*Burns:* Clinical studies have been conducted using DMSO on burn injuries. There are several properties unique to DMSO which have significant bearing on the healing process of the burned tissue and alleviating patient discomfort. DMSO is able to relieve a significant amount of pain within ten to thirty minutes after topical application. DMSO also has a tendency to cause a drying effect which helps prevent infection from developing in moist areas under burned tissue. Infection is the most serious complication of burn injury and in patients with extensive burns, it is the leading cause of death.

A study was conducted in Germany involving four patients with grade one and two burns (John and Laudahn, 1967). The patients received topical application of 2 to 5ml of 90 percent DMSO 2 to 4 times daily. Excellent results were observed in three patients and one patient received no benefits from the therapy.

Sehtman (1975) tested DMSO on burn patients in Argentina. Three patients with first- and second-degree burns were treated with DMSO with favorable response. Furthermore, these patients did not develop keloids, which are excessive scar tissue formations that frequently complicate the healing process. In this study, four patients were treated with DMSO on burn areas that had been grafted. The results on the graft patients were all excellent.

A further report by Engel (1967) reported DMSO treatment was effective in flattening burn scars that had already formed on ten patients with keloids.

Patients have also been treated with DMSO for sunburns and have experienced prompt pain relief of the burned areas of skin.

An animal study was conducted (Rosenbaum, et. al., 1967) treating burn eschars in rats with DMSO. It was found that DMSO prolonged survival after third-degree burns and enhanced the healing of the wounds.

Another animal study was conducted involving 38 rats to determine if skin treated with DMSO prior to an autograft survived better than the skin grafts not treated with DMSO. It was found that the DMSO decreased the skin's oxygen consumption by 29 percent and that these grafts had a 12 percent higher oxygen utilization than the freshly excised skin (Lessler, et. al., 1973).

**Cold injury**

*Cold Injury:* One of the initial medical uses of DMSO was in the preservation of cells exposed to low temperature; i.e., organs, spermatozoa, blood, and bone marrow. While, to date, few clinical trials have been conducted on the efficacy of DMSO in cold injury, there are scattered case histories of patients treated with DMSO for frostbite and other cold injuries.

A fifty-nine-year-old woman in Rockford, Illinois, had slipped and fallen on ice in front of her home at midnight. She was exposed to temperatures reaching 15 degrees below zero, Fahrenheit, for six hours before being taken to the hospital. Upon admission to the hospital, her rectal temperature was 16.6 degrees below normal. She was unresponsive and moved her frozen arms and legs fitfully. Her hands and feet were blue and both knees were bright red. Ice crystals were palpable in her knees, feet, and toes. She had no sensation in her discolored limbs. Her heartbeat was irregular.

Conventional treatment was initiated immediately in the intensive-care unit. By that evening, large blisters began forming on her toes and her fingers began to turn black.

At that time, a 65 percent solution of DMSO was applied to all extremities. Within ten minutes after application, the treated areas began to redden with the return of blood.

By the third day of treatment, sensation began returning to her toes and fingers, and by the seventh day she could flex the joints in her hands and feet. Treatment with DMSO continued for a month. At the end of treatment, all tissues were viable and sensation had completely returned to her extremities. Gangrene development and amputation had been averted by the use of DMSO.

**Recommended use of DMSO for cold injury**

For DMSO to be effective in cold injury, it must be applied within 12 hours following freezing. It is felt that after 24 hours, the damage sustained by the involved blood vessels might well be irreversible.

A study was conducted on rats subjected to frostbite. After injury, the rats were divided into groups and treated with warm water and 90 or 68.4 percent DMSO. The first two groups received no benefit; the frozen portions became gangrenous and fell off. However, the frozen tissue treated with 68.4 percent DMSO recovered completely. The most significant finding was that when either 90 or 68.4 percent DMSO was used to prevent frostbite damage, tissues so treated before injury remained undamaged by cold that had resulted in gangrene and amputation to untreated tissues (McGrady, 1973).

**Incision pain**

*Incision Pain:* Penrod, et. al., (1967) conducted a study on the effectiveness of DMSO on wounds of patients after surgery. The group of patients selected for the study had undergone chest surgery. This type of patient was selected because they often develop complications because they are unwilling to cough due to pain. After chest surgery, frequent coughing is necessary to clear the lungs of excess secretions and expand the lungs. A total of 24 patients were involved in the study. They were divided into three groups, one group given a 10 percent DMSO solution, a group given a 60 percent DMSO solution, and another group given an 80 percent concentration of DMSO. Ten ml of the DMSO was applied directly to the closed wound and to the area extending approximately ten inches on each side. This process was repeated every six hours for the first three days after surgery.

Early in the study it became quite apparent that the patients receiving the 60 and 80 percent DMSO received pain relief after each application. Furthermore, these two groups of patients were able to cough more effectively, move about more easily, resume motion of the shoulder and arm at an earlier stage, and enjoyed a less complicated and more rapid recovery course and required less narcotic medication for pain relief.

**Radiation injury**

*Radiation Injury:* Excessive radiation treatment of deep, malignant tumors also causes damage to the surrounding healthy tissue. Blistering of the skin surface, tissue erosion, dermatitis, itching, and pain, as well as fibrosis, a thickening of the underlying tissue, are frequent side effects of radiation therapy.

A study was conducted in Germany on the use of DMSO in the treatment and prevention of radiation tissue injury (Frommhold, Bublitz and Gries, 1967). This trial was conducted because of the positive results DMSO was having on scleroderma. In the disease process of scleroderma there are collagen or fibrotic changes occurring as are also present in a different manner in radiation-induced fibrosis.

The patients were treated with 90 percent DMSO applied to the irradiated area, as well as the surrounding tissue, and allowed to air dry. This procedure was repeated 2 to 3 times daily for a period of three to four months. The topical application of DMSO was generally tolerated well. A few patients noticed a slight burning or prickling sensation immediately following application.

The first positive effects of the treatment were manifested within five to eight days by a softening of the hardened, fibrotic tissues. This softening at the radiation site continued for 10 to 12 weeks. Furthermore, the patients treated with DMSO suffered fewer general untoward effects of radiation and obtained a speedier recovery.

**Eye disorders**

The first indication that DMSO would be therapeutic in eye disorders was discovered inadvertently. Certain patients with eye disorders who were receiving DMSO for other reasons felt their vision had improved also.

**Retinitis pigmentosa**

Investigation was begun in 1972 (Hill, 1975) following a rather spectacular recovery of vision by a patient suffering from retinitis pigmentosa. This patient received a topical application of 50 percent DMSO to the eye by eyecup immersion for 30 seconds twice daily. Prior to treatment, this patient had only been able to see hand motion with his right eye and the vision in his left eye was 20/200. After five days of treatment his vision was 20/70 in his left eye and he was able to count fingers at a five-foot distance. Furthermore, three months later, the vision in his left eye had improved to 20/50.

Hill (1981) investigated 19 patients over a five year period that were treated with DMSO for retinitis pigmentosa. The solution administered was one percent DMSO, five percent glycerin, and 0.5 percent superoxide dismutase dissolved in normal saline, filtered, and given in a dosage of one drop daily in each eye. The results showed 36 percent of the patients obtained visual acuity improvements; visual field improvement was noted in 16 percent. It was determined that DMSO had value in the treatment of retinal disease and that DMSO does not cause cataracts or other adverse eye effects.

An investigation conducted on 50 patients with retinitis pigmentosa and macular degeneration showed significant improvement was obtained in visual acuity, visual field, and night vision after DMSO therapy.

**DMSO and superoxide dismutase**

DMSO has been successfully used as a carrier for the enzyme superoxide dismutase in the treatment of various eye disorders such as macular edema and degenerative, traumatic endogenous and exogenous uvitis, and anterior, posterior, and cortical cataracts. The dosage employed is 5mg superoxide dismutase in 5ml of normal saline combined with 5ml of 25 percent DMSO, administered three times daily in each eye. DMSO is also effectively used to potentiate pilocarpine drugs used in open angle glaucoma when treatment with pilocarpine drugs alone does not bring satisfactory results.

**Ear, nose and throat disorders**

**Tinnitus**

*Tinnitus:* Tinnitus is a disorder of the ear in which the patient suffers from a variety of "ear noises." The noises are generally ringing, hissing, buzzing, or roaring in nature and very annoying. The disorder may be intermittent or constant and may often be accompanied by hearing loss. A possible cause of the disease is metabolic dysfunction induced by an alteration of blood circulation, vascular spasms, or possibly a tendency towards a diminished blood flow.

A study was conducted in Chile (Zuniga, 1975) on 15 patients who had suffered from tinnitus for a minimum of six months. The patients were treated for one month with DMSO combined with an anti-inflammatory and vasodilatory drug applied topically to the external canal of the ear in the form of a spray administered every four days. Further treatment with DMSO and a vasodilatory drug was administered daily in the form of an intramuscular injection.

After one month of treatment, the symptoms completely disappeared in nine patients and did not recur during one year of observation. Symptoms diminished in two patients and in four patients with permanent tinnitus, the symptoms recurred occasionally, generally triggered by exposure to cold weather.

A further significant finding during this study was that the temperature of the average patient's eardrum rose approximately one degree centigrade after treatment. This rise in temperature probably indicates improvement in the flow of blood to the inner ear.

**Acute otitis media**

*Otitis Media:* A therapeutic trial was conducted in Germany (Asen, 1967) on patients with acute otitis media, an inflammation of the middle ear. In 40 patients, one or two drops of DMSO and antibiotics were applied to the eardrum. A temporary burning sensation was observed by the patients treated. The results obtained were better when treatment was commenced early in the disease process. Rapid relief of pain following the treatment was attained. Excellent results were achieved in 16 patients, 18 patients noted improvement, and 6 patients showed no improvement following DMSO and antibiotic treatment.

**Chronic otitis media**

A similar study was conducted on 28 patients with chronic otitis media treated with DMSO and antibiotics. Excellent results were obtained with 4 patients, distinct improvement was achieved in 13 patients; however, these patients tended to relapse. Eleven patients experienced no improvement from the therapy. As these results indicate, the treatment was rather unsatisfactory. This could be largely due to the anatomy of the chronic ear inflammation.

**Eczymatous otitis and furnuncular otitis**

Further studies were conducted on 102 patients with eczymatous otitis and furnuncular otitis, which are very painful diseases of the ear canal. Considerable swelling is present and it is highly sensitive to pressure. The patients were treated with DMSO once or twice daily. The majority of the patients obtained very distinct pain regression after a few hours. Excellent results were obtained in 28 patients, 52 patients noted definite improvement, and 22 patients remained unimproved. The majority of the patients that did improve experienced remission of symptoms after only four applications of DMSO.

**Nose infections**

*Nose Infections:* Asen (1967) also treated 34 patients with various nose infections with DMSO. Excellent results were obtained in 16 patients, 15 patients noted improvement, and 3 patients experienced no improvement with DMSO therapy.

Throat and mouth infections

*Throat and Mouth Infections:* Studies were conducted on 119 patients with tonsillitis and pharangitis (Asen, 1967). External application resulted in occasional pain relief, but did not cause significant improvement. However, after direct application of DMSO or DMSO with antibiotics to the diseased area, 20 patients experienced excellent results, 72 patients noted improvement, and 27 observed no change.

Thirty-four patients were treated with DMSO for stomatitis aphthosa, a disease of the mouth where painful ulcers are present. Excellent results were obtained by 13 patients, 19 noted definite improvement, and 2 received no noticeable benefit. Generally, the best results were obtained after only two to four treatments. The swelling frequently disappeared within only a few hours.

Mental disorders

Mongolism

*Mongolism:* One of the many types of mental retardation is Down's Syndrome, commonly known as mongolism. This disorder is due to the trisomy of chromosome 21, which means that the cells contain three, rather than the normal two, twenty-first chromosomes.

The discovery of DMSO's ability to penetrate and diffuse without cellular alteration as well as its capacity to potentiate drugs taken with it awakened interest in using it as a vehicle in the treatment of mongolism and other retardation syndromes. The penetrating power of DMSO allows certain amino acids essential to nerve function (gama-aminobutyric acid, gama-amino-beta-hydroxybutyric acid, and acetylglutamine) to penetrate the meninges, the covering of the brain, and thus activate neurological functions that are suppressed in mental retardation syndromes.

Clinical studies were conducted in Chile with 64 mongoloid patients (Aspillaga, et. al., 1975). Half of the patients were controls; the remaining children were separated into two groups, those less than 3½ years of age, and those older.

The results of the study showed the DMSO-treated patients had significantly higher improvement than the controls in all areas—motor ability, speech, adaptation, and sociability. Interestingly, the younger group (3½ years old) showed greater improvement particularly in aspects of sociability and movement. The older children's scores were significantly improved in graphic age and movement. Furthermore, the older children also showed a rise in their intelligence quotient from the average of 29 to 40. The control group's I.Q. did not show an increase.

**Mental retardation**

*Mental Retardation:* A study was conducted in Oregon (Gabourie, et. al., 1975) on 67 children that were mentally retarded. This group of children manifested either Down's Syndrome, brain damage, or other types of retardation. Because a true double-blind study was impossible due to the inability to duplicate the DMSO odor in the control group, the "would have been" control children were given a low dosage of DMSO so the odor would be present in both groups.

The DMSO-treated group was given 0.10gm/kg body weight five times weekly for seven weeks, then 0.50gm/kg for seven weeks. The DMSO was added to orange juice and taken orally. During the study, there were two one-week breaks.

The children receiving the high dose of DMSO had 85 percent more gains in language, motor movement, and other psychometric areas than losses; the low dose group had 58 percent, and 22 percent in the group were not given any DMSO. Furthermore, the children taking high doses of DMSO showed a significantly higher age growth score than the other groups of children.

Another scientific team in Argentina (Giller and de Bernadou, 1975) tested DMSO in children mentally retarded due to various causes. The children were treated for 180 days or longer with DMSO-amino acid therapy. Prior to, during, and following the treatment, the children were tested in various areas of psychological and psychomotor growth. Highly significant progress was noted in all of the treated children, whereas in the control group there was hardly any variation noted. The team was studying a group of mongoloid babies who had been under treatment since their first month of life.

It has been suggested that some of the mental retardation patients might be further improved by combining intravenous DMSO and balanced nutrition with hyperbaric oxygen therapy. See Halstead (1980) for further details regarding hyperbaric oxygen therapy.

**Mental psychosis**

*Mental Psychosis:* In Peru a study was conducted (Ramirez and Luza, 1967) on 42 patients with mental disorders such as schizophrenia, manic depression, alcohol psychosis, anxiety, and neurosis. The patients were given DMSO intramuscularly two to three times daily. In the most disturbed patients, it was given up to five times daily.

**Schizophrenia**

Twenty-five schizophrenic patients were treated, and interestingly, the acute patients responded better than the chronic patients. Fourteen acute and four chronic patients reached complete remission and were discharged from the hospital. Results noted in the other groups tested were also significant as DMSO was noted to have an antipsychotic effect, decreasing agitation, restlessness, and anxiety symptoms. DMSO induced emotional calm followed by relief from psychotic and neurotic symptoms, but without the sedation of many tranquilizers.

**Disorders of the reproductive system**

**Female sterility**

*Female Sterility:* A study was conducted in Chile (Venegas, 1975) on 47 women who had been unable to become pregnant because of chronically inflamed Fallopian tubes. The Fallopian tubes are the passageways through which the ovum or egg passes from the ovary to the uterus. When these tubes become inflamed, the passageway is obstructed and pregnancy cannot occur.

The women were treated with a combination of DMSO, an antibiotic, a steroid, and an antihistamine that was injected into the Fallopian tubes every three days and was repeated six times. Initial examination of the tubes had been conducted prior to treatment and was repeated following treatment with the DMSO mixture. If, after three months of apparent good tubal function, pregnancy did not occur, the treatment was again repeated.

Pregnancy occurred in 27 of the 47 women treated. This success rate of 57 percent largely surpassed the results obtained by traditional treatment methods. In this study, DMSO was used as a drug potentiator, to assist tissue penetration of the drugs used, and as an anti-inflammatory agent.

**Envenomations**

A laboratory experiment was conducted on mice which had been injected with snake venom and DMSO. DMSO was found to enhance the envenomation process by decreasing the time required for the poison to kill and by rendering sublethal venom doses lethal. Subsequently the mice were injected with antivenin in combination with DMSO (Tiru-Chelvam, 1974). There was evidence that the venom lethality was enhanced by the administration of the DMSO-antivenin preparation as well. These two effects were paradoxical in that the venom lethality was enchanced while the antivenin had a lesser protective effect when combined with DMSO.

The mechanism of action by DMSO in envenomations is uncertain. The ability of DMSO to "transport" is probably only partially responsible, if at all. It appears that DMSO increases tissue permeability which passively enhances the distribution of venom.

# 6

# Answers To Commonly Asked Questions About DMSO

*Question: What is the best way to apply DMSO topically?*

Answer: Always, before applying DMSO, it is important to cleanse the skin area to be treated. If you are using a liquid preparation it can be applied with your fingertips or cotton-tip applicator. Another convenient way to apply it is with a small natural bristle paint or pastry brush. This prevents waste of the DMSO. Following application, allow the skin to dry for at least 20 minutes, after which the residual DMSO can be wiped off.

Generally, the DMSO cream or gel preparations tend to be more popular with patients because they are easier to apply; however, these media dilute the DMSO strength somewhat and therefore are slightly less effective.

*Question: I have noticed that the DMSO sold at hobby shops and flea markets tends to be cheaper than the DMSO available through my physician. Isn't all DMSO the same? Couldn't I safely obtain it from these cheaper sources?*

Answer: There are three grades of DMSO available on the market today. The analytical (spectroscope) grade is a highly purified form of

DMSO which is free of any particulate matter or contaminating agents. It is available in a 99.9 percent strength. The medical grade, available on a prescriptive basis, is free of any harmful contaminants and is generally available in 50 to 90 percent concentrations. The commercial grade is the grade most generally available, particularly from non-medical sources. This commercial grade DMSO can contain contaminants such as lead, cadmium, or other metals that may be harmful when used for medicinal purposes. Not all commercial grade DMSO contains contaminants; however, it is intended to be used as a solvent or in commercial use and the standards by which it is processed allow for the presence of contaminants.

The analytical grade DMSO is contaminant free. It is very important for anyone taking this grade to bear in mind that 99 percent strength DMSO should NEVER be taken topically or orally without dilution. This strength DMSO is much too powerful and can cause rashes and blisters on the skin. When using topical DMSO, the strength should generally be from 70 to 90 percent, depending on the tolerance of the patient. The concentration should never exceed 90 percent in topical application.

Contaminants such as bacteria cannot grow in any grade DMSO that is at or above a 25 percent strength. However, one must bear in mind there are other harmful contaminants possibly present in inferior grades.

*Question: I was given DMSO by my physician to use on bursitis in my shoulder. After the first application I noticed the area under my arm where the DMSO had also been applied was very reddened whereas the shoulder area was not. What caused this to occur?*

Answer: There are various areas of skin on the body that are very sensitive, such as the face, neck, and underarms. When using DMSO on these areas, it is best to use a more dilute concentration. Begin with a 70 percent solution and increase to your tolerance level. You will probably notice that even though only the 70 percent DMSO is tolerated by these areas initially, after a few days the higher concentrations can be applied without the redness and discomfort noticed at the onset of DMSO treatment. It has been found that not only are different skin areas more sensitive to DMSO, but certain people respond differently. Very light complexioned people and redheads tend to tolerate the lower concentrations (70 percent) of DMSO only.

*Question: I applied some DMSO to my left elbow because of severe pain I was experiencing due to arthritis. It didn't seem to help. Do you know why?*

Answer: Due to the nature of arthritis, the results obtained by DMSO are frequently not immediate. Treatment of the affected area must be repeated and consistent for optimal results. It should be remembered as well that in some patients certain types of arthritis are unresponsive to DMSO treatment.

Another thing to remember in the topical application of DMSO is to always apply it not only to the affected area, but also to a large area surrounding it. For instance, when applying DMSO to your elbow, apply it approximately six inches above and below. Allow it to dry for about 20 minutes, then remove any residual DMSO with a cloth or tissue. This process can be repeated three or four times daily if necessary. Remember, for optimal results a 70 to 90 percent concentration should be used.

*Question: When I apply DMSO to my arthritic finger joints the pain goes away; however, the pain returns within three or four hours. How often can I repeat the application?*

Answer: Generally, DMSO can be applied every four to six hours when necessary. However, it is best to always consult your prescribing physician in order to determine your optimal dosage.

*Question: When I apply DMSO on my skin I get a slight burning sensation. Do I have an allergy to it or is this to be expected?*

Answer: This burning or tingling sensation that often occurs when utilizing higher concentrations of DMSO is caused by a local histamine-releasing action at the site of application. This minor side effect frequently disappears after several applications and does not necessarily indicate an allergy to DMSO.

*Question: DMSO has such a potent, bitter taste. What is the easiest way to take it by mouth?*

Answer: There is no easy way to take DMSO orally, but do not attempt to take it undiluted. The taste can be subdued by adding it to one half glass of milk or orange juice. Some patients say it is easier to use when something tart is taken along with it, such as a pickle or a green olive.

*Question: I have heard DMSO can take harmful substances into the skin. I apply DMSO to my arthritic toes. Should I wash it off before putting on my hose?*

Answer: The DMSO need not be washed off before putting on your hose. However, it is important to allow the DMSO to dry completely before putting your hose on. DMSO can dissolve certain types of synthetic hose, rayons, polyvinyl chlorides, polyurethanes, methacrylates, and acrylics. DMSO is generally not a solvent for cotton, wool, leather, nylon, and polyester at room temperature. Also one should use caution when bringing DMSO into contact with textile dyes because they may penetrate the skin.

*Question: I have been using DMSO for headaches by applying it to my forehead. Should the DMSO get into my eyes, would this cause harmful side effects?*

Answer: It is not harmful for small amounts of DMSO to get into the eye. Actually, for some eye diseases, dilute amounts of DMSO (12 to 15 percent) are used as treatment. It should be noted that when DMSO is instilled into the eye or gets into the eye by accident, there might be a slight burning sensation for 15 to 20 seconds. This should not cause alarm and will go away quite rapidly. DMSO should not be purposely placed in the eye without the advice of an experienced physician.

*Question: Is there anything that can be done about the breath and body odor that accompanies the use of DMSO?*

Answer: This is one of the natural end results in the systemic metabolism of DMSO; it is apparent in the majority of patients using it. To avoid this, it is helpful to take a shower at least once a day and wash your hair frequently. The odor is present in the oil and sweat glands, but is most evident on the breath. At the present time, extensive research is being conducted in an attempt to determine a method for overcoming this objectionable side effect. Results of some studies in this area have shown that urea may greatly reduce the odor of topically applied DMSO. It also appears that a Swiss pharmaceutical firm has produced an odorless DMSO, but unfortunately is not allowed to distribute it in the U.S.

*Question: Another physician has prescribed sleeping pills for me which I use occasionally when traveling. Will the DMSO have an effect on my response to the sleeping pills?*

Answer: DMSO does potentiate the action of many drugs including sleeping pills and pain medication. To be safe, it is important to consult a physician that is familiar with the action of DMSO prior to using it in conjunction with any other drug.

*Question: What are some of the adverse side effects I should watch for while taking DMSO?*

Answer: The most common side effect, an almost universal side effect, is the objectionable breath odor. Other side effects, particularly when taking very high doses of DMSO, are occasional headaches, nausea, or dizziness. When DMSO is applied to the skin, a local skin rash occasionally results. If a high concentration of DMSO is taken, about 80 or 90 percent, skin dryness and possible skin flaking frequently occurs. This condition can be alleviated by application of *Aloe vera*, jojoba oil, or a vitamin E cream preparation after the DMSO application has dried. Always bear in mind that a cream preparation containing chemicals or perfumes should not be used since these substances can be drawn into the skin by DMSO.

*Question: For years I have had severe pain in my right knee. I have used DMSO topically at the site of discomfort and the pain has been greatly reduced. However, I have had silicone implanted in my knee joint. Will the DMSO have an effect on the silicone?*

Answer: DMSO does not affect silicone implants, nor will it have an adverse effect on implanted pins or valves.

*Question: I have been told that you should be able to taste DMSO after it is applied to the skin. I have never been able to taste it. Does this mean my body does not absorb it or that it is not working for me?*

Answer: Each patient has a slightly different metabolism and reacts to DMSO in his own unique way. Some patients are not able to taste the DMSO and a rare few will exhibit no breath odor after taking it. This in no way means DMSO is not working for you.

*Question: I have heard that if a patient takes DMSO over a long period of time, eye disorders such as cataracts or blindness could result. Is this true?*

Answer: No. Eye disorders do not occur. This is a frequent misconception that is prevalent among the poorly informed professionals. In three animal species not closely related to primates or man, refractory lens changes did occur when these animals were given 100 times the average human dosage. These eye changes have never occurred in man and need not cause concern.

*Question: I have heard that DMSO is illegal everywhere except Oregon, Florida, and Louisiana. Do I have to go there to obtain it?*

Answer: The FDA approved prescriptive DMSO for human treatment in 1978. The approval was for the treatment of interstitial cystitis, a rare bladder disease. However, once a drug is approved by the FDA for any condition, a physician in the United States is free to prescribe it for whatever illness he feels it is appropriate.

*Question: I heard through a friend that one can take his daily dosage of DMSO in an injection if taking it orally is too objectionable. Is this done?*

Answer: DMSO can safely be administered intravenously or intramuscularly. It would be best to consult your physician to see whether this route of administration is warranted in your case. When DMSO is administered either into the vein or muscle, the dosage strength should not exceed 20 percent or local tissue damage could result. Furthermore, unless the DMSO is combined with an anesthetic, such as xylocaine, it can be quite painful when given intramuscularly.

# 7

# The Question of Legality

The legal status of DMSO is a subject that is grossly misunderstood by both physicians and laymen. Much of this confusion has been generated by the legal gyrations and a blizzard of "white papers" and "fact sheets" released by the United States Food and Drug Administration. The legal benchmarks for the approved uses of DMSO are as follows:

**Legal status of DMSO**

DMSO therapy in humans was started by Stanley W. Jacob, M.D., and his associates about 1961 at the University of Oregon Medical School. By late 1965, an estimated 100,000 patients had used DMSO for the treatment of sprains, bruises, and minor burns. Most of this work had been conducted under the usual FDA Investigational New Drug Applications (IND's).

When toxicological studies showed that DMSO altered the refractive index of the lens of eyes in experimental animals the FDA terminated all clinical research on November 11, 1965. This termination order was made despite the fact there was no clinical evidence that refractive index changes occurred in humans.

**Termination of use**

**Limited use resumed**

In December 1966, the FDA permitted a limited resumption of clinical testing of DMSO in the United States.

The FDA published a further revision of its DMSO policy in September 1968, permitting topical application to the skin for not more than 14 days for less serious disabilities, such as acute musculoskeletal conditions. This permission was based on a toxicological study in humans that provided no evidence of eye toxicity due to DMSO in humans during short-term topical use. However, this decision was tempered by additional animal studies which demonstrated that prolonged use of DMSO in animals caused lens opacities. Nevertheless, there was still no evidence that lens toxicities had ever occurred in humans.

**NAS-NRC evaluates safety**

Then, in 1972, the FDA provided the National Academy of Sciences—National Research Council (Division of Medical Sciences) with a contract (FDA 70-22, Task Order No. 14) to provide the FDA with an evaluation of the safety and efficacy of DMSO therapy in humans. The final report of the NAS-NRC was released in August 1973. The NAS-NRC selected a blue-ribbon panel of "experts" who were "chosen because of recognized scholarly competence and due consideration for the balance of disciplines appropriate to the project." The members of the committee reviewed about 1,200 papers on DMSO in the domestic and foreign literature and 193 volumes of reports that had been submitted to the FDA by manufacturers and independent investigators.

**NAS-NRC study questioned**

Although this FDA contract evaluation appeared to be an impressive scientific undertaking, it amounted to merely a review of the existing literature by a panel of inexperienced individuals who had little or no personal laboratory or clinical experience with DMSO. Dr. Stanley Jacob, who is unquestionably the world's leading authority on DMSO, was not even selected as a member of the panel. However, the "experts" did allow him to make an appearance and to submit his views on the subject, some of which appeared to have been largely disregarded. There were several conclusions by the NAS-NRC panel which are especially noteworthy.

NAS-NRC conclusions

*"DMSO produces side effects, particularly in the skin, in most persons treated and there have been sporadic cases in which DMSO has, with reasonable confidence, been linked to acute generalized urticaria in man. There is also evidence that in some species of laboratory animals DMSO in doses somewhat higher than those contemplated for man produces a unique alteration of the lens. The nature of these side effects, the import of the animal data, and the incidence of adverse reactions alone would not warrant withholding the drug in clinical circumstances in which it gave promise of saving life or in which it would clearly be more effective than currently available treatment in arresting a disease process, reducing disability, or relieving pain.*

*"The nature of the evidence of effectiveness of DMSO is not such as to warrant the release of the drug for prescription in general medical practice at this time. There is suggestive evidence that DMSO may be effective in the treatment of acute traumatic injury and nontraumatic painful shoulder and in relieving the pain of rheumatoid arthritis. Some investigators have claimed that DMSO may be superior to currently available forms of treatment in cutaneous scleroderma and in interstitial cystitis, but the evidence does not allow a conclusion to be drawn in that respect. As a vehicle, DMSO may enhance the effect of other therapeutic agents such as fungicides and antiviral agents.*

Restriction of use recommended

*"In view of the toxicity and lack of demonstrated efficacy in prior studies, the use of the drug should be restricted to investigational circumstances until it can be clearly demonstrated in some clinical condition that its therapeutic effect warrants the attendant side effects.*

*"More reliable data are needed on the toxicity of DMSO and on its mechanism of action."*

In brief, the NAS-NRC panel of inexperienced "experts" essentially confirmed the position of the FDA, which is what they wanted to hear. To the credit of the panel, they felt that the published criteria for acceptance of individual applications for clinical investigation of DMSO was "overly restrictive."

**True double-blind studies impossible**

One of the concerns of this panel was the inability of an investigator to find another substance that was capable of producing the unique side effects of DMSO, namely, the garlicky breath odor and skin irritation. Failure to find a suitable DMSO placebo eliminated any opportunity for conducting true double-blind studies. The NAS-NRC is of particular significance because it provided a biopolitical basis for some of the subsequent legal actions of the FDA.

**FDA approval for interstitial cystitis**

In 1978, after a struggle of more than a decade, the FDA finally approved the prescriptive use of DMSO for the treatment of interstitial cystitis, a rare bladder disease.

**Application for scleroderma refused**

In early 1980, on the advice of its Arthritis Advisory Committee, the FDA refused an application for marketing DMSO for the treatment of cutaneous ulcers in scleroderma.

At present, the FDA is not requiring monitoring of the eyes in investigational studies in which topical exposure to DMSO is limited to 14 days or less. However, the FDA continues to contend that present studies are insufficient at this time to determine whether prolonged use of DMSO in high doses in humans poses a risk of ocular damage.

**Physicians not limited by suggested use of drugs**

Many physicians are apparently oblivious to the fact that the Sherman Food, Drug and Cosmetic Law does not prevent a physician from prescribing a drug for a condition not specified in the drug manufacturer's advertising which was approved in a Federal or State New Drug Application. This matter was clearly defined in the decision by the U.S. Federal District Court for the Middle District of Alabama,

**USA vs H. Ray Evers, M.D.**

Northern Division, in the case of the United States of America vs. H. Ray Evers, M.D., Civil Action No. 78-93-N, dated 27 June, 1978. The case was spearheaded against Dr. Evers by the Food and Drug Administration and alleged: (1) that Dr. Evers had been engaged in promoting and administering EDTA in the treatment of arteriosclerosis; (2) that the labeling of the drug, namely the package insert, which is prescribed and approved by the FDA, indicated the drug is recommended for treatment of heavy metal poisoning, but not for the treatment of arteriosclerosis; (3) that patients treated by Dr. Evers were being subjected to an unwarranted risk of grave physical injury or death as a result of the treatment; and (4) that the promotion and administration of EDTA amounted to mislabeling of the drug in violation of interstate commerce regulations. Dr. Evers contended that he was a licensed physician in the State of Alabama, and that as a licensed physician he has the right and a duty to use and prescribe drugs which in the opinion of the physician are in the best interests of the patient. Dr. Evers also contended that the FDA does not prohibit a licensed physician using a drug for a disease in a patient in any manner which is not contraindicated on the package insert.

**FDA attempts to restrain use of EDTA**

The FDA attempted to obtain an injunction restraining: (1) the receipt or possession of EDTA, or any other chelating agent; (2) the continuance of administration of chelation therapy by Dr. Evers; and (3) the allowance of regular inspection of Dr. Ever's clinic by the FDA.

The Court established the fact that the legal issue in this case was the question of whether a licensed physician may be enjoined from prescribing for his patients a drug of which the package insert is silent as to whether the drug is indicated or contraindicated for the patient's illness.

It is interesting to note that irrespective of the strong medical school of thought that chelation has not been clinically shown to help arteriosclerosis, the weight of the

**Arteriosclerosis and chelation therapy**

evidence submitted to the Court was to the contrary. The Court was further of the opinion that there is a school of thought among medical experts in the United States and foreign countries that arteriosclerosis may be satisfactorily treated with chelation therapy, that the risks when the therapy is properly administered to select patients are minimal, and that in many cases the probable benefits outweigh the probable risks in such treatment.

**Legal restrictions on medical profession declined**

The Court noted that the U.S. Congress did not intend the Food and Drug Administration to interfere with medical practice as between the physician and the patient. Congress recognized a patient's right to seek civil damages in the courts if there should be evidence of malpractice, and declined to provide any legislative restrictions upon the medical profession. It appeared to the Court that such a restriction would exceed the powers of Congress.

**Court defends "best judgment" of physicians**

The Court further stated that "when physicians go beyond the directions given in the package insert it does not mean they are acting illegally or unethically and Congress did not intend to empower the FDA to interfere with medical practice by limiting the ability of physicians to prescribe according to their best judgment. See FDA Consumer, November 1975, p. 7." It was the decision of the Court that Dr. Evers was not misbranding the drug in question, and therefore denied the relief prayed by the plaintiff.

The sum and substance of the Federal Court decision in the Ray Evers case is this: Once the FDA has approved a drug, for whatever purpose, it is the prerogative of the physician to determine the clinical application of the drug, its route of administration, and its dosage. The FDA is not licensed to practice medicine in any state in the United States and they have no legal jurisdiction as to how a licensed physician administers an approved drug.

**"Food and Drug Reform Act of 1979"**

There is now a bill (HR 54) in the United States Congress entitled "Food and Drug Reform Act of 1979" introduced by Representative Steven D. Symms (Idaho) providing for a major reformation of the existing food and drug laws. A reform of the entire operations of the FDA, especially their regulatory powers, is long overdue.

# References


Adamson, J. E., Horton, C. E., Crawford, H. H., and W. T. Ayers, 1966. The effects of dimethyl sulfoxide on the experimental pedicle flap: A preliminary report. Plast. and Reconstruct. Surg., 37:105-110.

Armstrong, J. R., and I. Cohn, 1967. The influence of DMSO on intraperitoneal implantation of tumor cells. Ann. N.Y. Acad. Sci. 141(1):221-224.

Asen, H., 1967. Dimethyl sulfoxide: A new concept in the treatment of ENT diseases. Ann. N.Y. Acad. Sci. 141(1):451-456.

Ashwood-Smith, M. J. 1961. Inability of dimethyl sulphoxide to protect mouse testes against the effect of x-radiation. Intern. J. Radiation Biol. 3:101.

Ashwood-Smith, M. J., 1961. The radioprotective action of dimethyl sulfoxide and various other sulfoxides. Intern. J. Radiation Biol. 3:41-48.

Ashwood-Smith, M. J., 1967. Radioprotective and cryoprotective properties of dimethyl sulfoxide in cellular systems. Ann. N.Y. Acad. Sci. 141(1):45-62.

Ashwood-Smith, M. J., 1971. Radioprotective and cryoprotective properties of DMSO. In: Dimethyl sulfoxide, basic concepts of DMSO. Vol. 1 (Eds. S. W. Jacob, E. E. Rosenbaum, and D. C. Wood), Marcel Dekker, Inc., New York, pp. 147-187.

Ashwood-Smith, M. J., 1975. Current concepts concerning radioprotective and cryoprotective properties of dimethyl sulfoxide in cellular systems. Ann. N.Y. Acad. Sci. 243:246-256.

Aspillaga, M. J., Morizon, G., Avendano, I., Sanchez, M. and L. Capdeville, 1975. Dimeth sulfoxide therapy in severe retardation in mongoloid children. Ann. N.Y. Acad. Sci. 243:421-431.

Astley, J. P. and M. Levine, 1975. Effect of dimethyl sulfoxide on permeability of human skin in vitro. J. Pharm. Sci. 65(2):210-215.

Ayre, J. E., and J. LeGuerrier, 1967. Some (regressive) effects of DMSO dexamethasone upon cervical cells in cervical dysplagia and carcinoma in situ. Ann. N.Y. Acad. Sci. 141(1):414-422.

Baker, H., 1968. The effects of dimethylsufloxide dimethylformamide and dimethylacetamide on the cutaneous barrier to water in human skin. J. Invest. Dermatol. 50(4):283-288.

Barnett, B. M., 1972. Radioprotective effects of dimethyl sulfoxide in drosophila melanogaster. Radiation Res. 51:134.

Barnett, K. C. and P. R. B. Noel, 1967. Dimethyl sulphoxide and lens changes in primates. Nature. 214:1115-1116.

Bartfield, H. and A. Goldstein, 1975. Cell-mediated immunity: Its modulation by dimethyl sulfoxide. Ann. N.Y. Acad. Sci. 243:81-90.

Bayare, A. A., Dubinski, M. B. and A. A. Skager, 1971. Experiment in the application of dymethylsulfoxide (DMSO) in the treatment of purulent diseases. Paper presented at the IX Scientific Conference of Surgeons and Anesthesiologists of the Estonian. Soviet Union.

Bergreen, L., 1980. The strange saga of a painkiller. T.V. Guide 28(30):2-6.

Bernath, Z., Chacon, E., Bennett, N. and A. Rivera, 1980. Clinical experience in the treatment of the asthmatic syndrome with a combination of simesuline, 1, 3 dimethyl xanthine-ethylene diamine, chlorpheniramine, and an anti-inflammatory. Unpublished data.

Birkmayer, W., Panielczyk, W. and H. Werner, 1966. Zur wirkung von DMSO auf die blutgerinnung. In: Dimethylsulfoxyd—DMSO. Internationales Symposium. (Eds. G. Laundahn and K. Gertich), Wein. Saladruck., Berlin. pp. 144-149.

Block, L. H., 1964. Dimethyl sulfoxide. Medicinal and pharmaceutical aspects. Drug. Cosmet. Ind., 95(3):342-465.

Blumenthal, L. S. and M. Fuchs, 1967. The clinical use of dimethyl sulfoxide on various headaches, musculoskeletal and other general medical disorders. Ann. N.Y. Acad. Sci. 141(1):572-585.

Borenfreund, E., Steinglass, M., Korngold, G. and A. Bendich, 1975. Effect of dimethyl sulfoxide and dimethylformamide on the growth and morphology of tumor cells. Ann. N.Y.

Acad. Sci. 243:164-171.

Bradham, G. B. and J. J. Sample, 1967. The vascular and thermal effects of dimethyl sulfoxide. Ann. N.Y. Acad. Sci. 141(1): 225-230.

Brechner, V. L., Cohen, D. D. and I. Pretsky, 1967. Dermal anesthesia by the topical application of tetracaine base dissolved in dimethyl sulfoxide. Ann. N.Y. Acad. Sci. 141(1):524.531.

Brink, J. J. and D. G. Stein, 1967. Premoline levels in brain enhancement by dimethyl sufloxide. Science, 158:1479.

Brobyn, R. D., 1975. The human toxicology of dimethyl sulfoxide. Ann. N.Y. Acad. Sci. 243:497-506.

Brown, J. H., 1967. Clinical experience with DMSO in acute musculoskeletal conditions comparing a noncontrolled series with a controlled double blind study. Ann. N.Y. Acad. Sci. 141(1):495-505.

Brown, V. K., Robinson, J. and D. E. Stevenson, 1963. A note on the toxicity and solvent properties of dimethyl sulfoxide. J. Pharm. Pharmacol. 15:688-692.

Caldwell, A. D. S., Bye, P. G. T. and M. H. Briggs, 1967. Side effects of dimethyl sulphoxide. Nature, 215:1168.

Caujolle, F. and D. Meyner, 1957. L'indice d' agressivite' (DL 50 limite). Bull. Acad. Med., 17:362.

Caujolle, F., Caujolle, D. Bouissou, H. and M. M. Calvet, 1964. Toxicite' et aptitudes pharmacologiques du DMSO. Comptes rendus. 258:2224.

Caujolle, M. F., Caujolle, D., Cross, S., Calvet, M. and Y. Tollon, 1965. Pouvoir teratogene du dimethylsulfoxyde et du diethylsulfoxyde. C. R. Acad. Sci. Paris. 260(12):327-330.

Caujolle, F. M. E., Caujolle, D. H., Cros, S. B., and M. M. J. Calvet, 1967. Limits of toxic and teratogenic tolerance of DMSO. Ann. N.Y. Acad. Sci. 141(1):110-126.

Ching-jung, C. and L. Hsi-shun, 1975. Effect of topical use of comptothecine-dimethyl sulfoxide solution in psoriasis. Chin. Med. J. 1(5):355-360.

Conover, T. E., 1975. Influence of nonionic organic solutes on various reactions of energy conservation and utilization. Ann. N.Y. Acad. Sci. 243:24-37.

Cornejo, J. G. and R. E. Lagos, 1975. Dimethyl sulfoxide therapy as toxicity-reducing agent and potentiator of cyclophosphamide in the treatment of different types of cancer. Ann. N.Y. Acad. Sci. 243:412-420.

Cowie, J. M. G. and P. M. Toporowski, 1961. Association in the binary liquid system, dimethylsulphoxide-water. Can. J. Chem. 39:2240.

Crown Zellerbach Corporation, 1980. Dimethyl sulfoxide technical bulletin. Chemical Products Div., Camas, Washington, 28p.

David, N. A., 1972. The pharmacology of dimethyl sulfoxide. A. Rev. Pharmac. 12:353-374.

Demos, C. H., Beckloff, G. L., Donin, M. N. and P. M. Oliver, 1967. Dimethyl sulfoxide in musculoskeletal disorders. Ann. N.Y. Acad. Sci. 141(1):516.523.

Denko, C. W., Goodman, R. M., Miller, R. and T. Donovan, 1967. Distribution of dimethyl sulfoxide —$^{35}$S in the rat. Ann. N.Y. Acad. Sci. 141(1):77-84.

Dennis, A. J. and H. E. Wilson, 1975. Altered mitogenic responsiveness of chronic leukemic lymphocytes and normal human lymphocytes treated with dimethyl sulfoxide. Ann. N.Y. Acad. Sci. 243:73-80.

DiStefano, V. and H. H. Borgstedt, 1964. Reduction of dimethylsulfoxide to dimethylsulfide in the cat. Science, 144:1137-1138.

DiStefano, V. and J. J. Klahn, 1965. Observations on the pharmacology and hemolytic activity of dimethyl sulfoxide. Toxicol. Appl. Pharmacol. 7:660-666.

Dodd, J. L. and J. Sherwell, 1968. Local Protection against x-irradiation by DMSO. Brit. J. Radiol. 41:950.

Dubinsky, M. B. and A. A. Skager, 1975. Experience in the use of dimethyl sulfoxide in the diseases of the supporting motor apparatus and general supportive surgery. Ann. N.Y. Acad. Sci. 243:494-496.

Embery, G. and P. H. Dungard, 1971. The isolation of dimethyl sulfoxide soluble components from human epidermal preparations: A possible mechanism of action of dimethyl sulfoxide in effecting percutaneous migration phenomena. J. Invest. Dermatol. 57(5): 308-311.

Engel, M. F., 1967. Indications and contraindications for the use of DMSO in clinical dermatology. Ann. N.Y. Acad. Sci. 141(1):638-645.

Farrant, J., 1964. Pharmacological actions and toxicity of dimethyl sulphoxide and other compounds which protect smooth muscle during freezing and thawing. J. Pharm. Pharmacol. 16:472-483.

FDA, 1980. Use of DMSO for unapproved indications. FDA Drug Bul. 10(3):20-21.

Finney, J. W., Urschel, H. C., Balla, G. A., Race, G. J., Jay, B. E., Pingree, H. P., Dorman, H. L. and J. T. Mallams, 1967. Protection of the ischemic heart with DMSO alone or DMSO with hydrogen peroxide. Ann. N.Y. Acad. Sci. 141(1):231-241.

Fishman, E. G., Jenkins, L. J., Coon, R. A. and R. A. Jones, 1969. Effects of acute and repeated inhalation of dimethyl sulfoxide in rats. Toxic Appl. Pharmac 15:74-82.

Fletcher, W. S. and D. L. Dennis, 1967. The effect of DMSO on the induction of breast cancer in the rat. Ann. N.Y. Acad. Sci. 141(1): 214-220.

Formanek, K. and W. Kovak, 1966. Die wirkung von DMSO auf experimentell erzeugte rattenpfotenodem. In: Dimethylsulfoxyd—DMSO. Internationales Symposium. Wein. Saladruck., Berlin. pp. 18-21.

Formanek, K. and R. Suckert, 1966. Diuretische wirkung von DMSO. In: Dimethylsulfoxyde—DMSO. Internationales Symposium. Wein. Saladruck., Berlin. pp. 21-24.

Frommhold, W., Bublitz, G. and G. Gries, 1967. The use of DMSO for the treatment of postirradiation subcutaneous plaques. Ann. N.Y. Acad. Sci. 141(1):603-612.

Gabourie, J., Becker, J. W., Batemen, B., Dunn, M. and S. Jacob, 1975. Oral dimethyl sulfoxide in mental retardation. Ann. N.Y. Acad. Sci. 243:449-459.

Gandiha, A. and I. G. Marshall, 1972. Some actions of dimethylsulphoxide at the neuromuscular junction. J. Pharm. Pharmacol. 24:417-419.

Giller, A. and M. E. M. de Bernadou, 1975. Dimethyl sulfoxide therapy in nonmongoloid infantile oligophrenia. Ann. N.Y. Acad. Sci. 243:432-448.

Goldman, L. and K. W. Kitzmiller, 1965. Topical 5-iodo-2'-deoxyuridine in dimethylsulfoxide (DMSO). A new treatment for severe herpes simplex. Ohio Med. J. 61:532-533.

Golomazov, M. F., 1970. Clinical morphological characteristics of the healing of purulent wounds under the effects of dimethylsulfoxide. Klim. Khir. (Kisv), 2:52-57.

Gordon, D. M., 1967. Dimethyl sulfoxide in ophthalmology, with especial reference to possible toxic effects. Ann. N.Y. Acad. Sci. 141(1):392-401.

Gordon, D. M. and K. E. Kleberger, 1968. The effect of dimethyl sulfoxide (DMSO) on animal and human eyes. Arch. Ophthal. 79:423-427.

Görög, P. and I. B. Kovacs, 1968. Effect of dimethyl sulfoxide (DMSO) on various experimental inflammations. Curr. Ther. Res. 10:486-492.

Görög, P. and I. B. Kovacs, 1975. Antiarthritic and antithrombotic effects of topically applied dimethyl sulfoxide. Ann. N.Y. Acad. Sci. 243:91-97.

Graham, W. P., 1975. A comparison of glycerol and dimethyl sulfoxide as cryoprotective agents for an experimental tumor: A pilot study. Ann. N.Y. Acad. Sci. 243:317-319.

Gries, G., Bublitz, G. and J. Lindner, 1967. The effect of dimethyl sulfoxide on the components of connective tissue (clinical and experimental investigations). Ann. N.Y. Acad. Sci. 141(1):630-637.

Halstead, B. W., 1978. Amygdalin (laetrile) therapy. Golden Quill, Colton, 47 p.

Halstead, B. W., 1979. Chelation therapy patient handbook. Golden Quill, Colton, 22 p.

Halstead, B. W., 1980. Hyperbaric oxygen therapy. Golden Quill, Colton, 26 p.

Halstead, B. W., 1980. The scientific basis of EDTA chelation therapy. Golden Quill, Colton, 113 p.

Hamaguchi, K., 1964. Effect of dimethyl sulfoxide on the stability of muramidase. J. Biochem. (Tokyo), 56:441.

Hamar, D. W., Huang, S. and F. C. Chow, 1974. Effect of alanine and dimethyl sulfoxide on the solubility of calcium phosphate, magnesium phosphate and caldium oxalate. Biochem. Med. 11(1):98-102.

Hanig, J. P., Morrison, J. M. and S. Krop, 1971. Increase of blood-brain barrier permeability to catecholamines by dimethyl sulphoxide in the neonate chick. J. Pharm. Pharmacol. 23:386-387.

Henderson, T. R., Henderson, R. F. and J. L. York, 1975. Effects of dimethyl sulfoxide on subunit proteins. Ann. N.Y. Acad. Sci. 243:38-53.

Herschler, R. J. and S. W. Jacob, 1970. Therapeutic administration of effective amounts of dimethyl sulfoxide to human and animal subjects. U.S. Pat. No. 3,549,770:1-34.

Herschler, R. and S. W. Jacob, 1980. The case of dimethyl sulfoxide. In: Controversies in therapeutics (Ed. L. Lasagna). W. B. Saunders Co., Philadelphia, pp. 519-529.

Herzmann, E., 1968. Studies on the effect of dimethyl sulfoxide on experimental hypercholesteremia in young cocks. Acta. Biol. Med. Ger. 20:483.

Hill, R. V., 1975. Dimethyl sulfoxide in the treatment of retinal disease. Ann. N.Y. Acad. Sci. 243:485-490.

Hill, R. V., 1981. Personal Communication.

Hixson, G. F., 1955. Report on laboratory vitamin technology, M543. Stephan Chemical Co., 15 p.

Horita, A. and L. J. Weber, 1964. Skin penetrating property of drugs dissolved in dimethylsulfoxide (DMSO) and other vehicles. Life Sci. 3:1389-1395.

Hucker, H. B., Ahmad, P. M. and E. A. Miller, 1965. Physiological disposition and metabolism of dimethyl sulfoxide (DMSO). Federation Proc. 24:546.

Hucker, H. B., Ahmad, P. M. and E. A. Miller, 1966. Absorption, distribution, and metabolism of dimethylsulfoxide in the rat, rabbit, and guinea pig. J. Pharmacol. Exp. Therap. 154:176-184.

Hucker, H. B., Ahmad, P. M., Miller, E. A. and R. Brobyn, 1966. Metabolism of dimethyl sulfoxide to dimethyl sulfone in the rat and man. Nature, 209:619-620.

Hucker, H. B., Miller, J. K., Hochberg, A., Brobyn, R. D., Riordan, F. H. and B. Calesnick, 1967. Studies on the absorption, excretion, and metabolism of dimethylsulfoxide (DMSO) in man. J. Pharmacol. Exp. Ther. 155(2): 309-317.

Hull, F. W., Wood, D. C. and R. D. Brobyn, 1969. Eye effects of DMSO. Report of negative results. N.W. Medicine. 68:39-41.

Jacob, S. W., 1965. Dimethyl sulfoxide, its basic pharmacology and usefulness in the therapy of headaches. Headache 5:78-81.

Jacob, S. W., 1966. Dimethyl sulfoxide (DMSO) —a new concept in surgery. Amer. J. Surg. 111:160.

Jacob, S. W., 1969. DMSO: potential usefulness in physical therapy. Phys. Ther. 49(5):470-475.

Jacob, S. W., 1969. Dimethyl sulfoxide (DMSO) —current concepts in toxicology, pharmacology, and clinical usefulness in surgery. Amer. J. Surg. 35(8):564-573.

Jacob, S. W., 1971. Pharmacology of DMSO. In: Dimethyl sulfoxide, basic concepts of DMSO. Vol. 1 (Eds. S. W. Jacob, E. E. Rosenbaum and D. C. Wood), Marcel Dekker, Inc., New York, pp. 99-112.

Jacob, S. W., 1979. Personal Communication.

Jacob, S. W., 1980. Current status of DMSO. American Academy of Medical Preventics Convention. Reno, Nevada (unpublished).

Jacob, S. W., Bischel, M. and R. J. Herschler, 1964. Dimethyl sulfoxide: Effects on the permeability of biologic membranes (preliminary report). Curr. Ther. Res. 6(3):193-198.

Jacob, S. W. and R. Herschler, 1975. Biological actions of dimethyl sulfoxide. Ann. N.Y. Acad. Sci. 243:1-510.

Jacob, S. W. and E. E. Rosenbaum, 1966. The toxicology of dimethyl sulfoxide (DMSO). Headache 6:127-136.

Jacob, S. W. and D. C. Wood, 1967. Notes on dimethyl sulfoxide symposium: Vienna, Austria, November 8 and 9, 1966. Curr. Ther. Res. 9(4):229-233.

Jacob, S. W. and D. C. Wood, 1967. Dimethyl sulfoxide (DMSO) toxicology, pharmacology and clinical experience. Am. J. Surg. 114: 414-426.

Jacob, S. W. and D. C. Wood, 1971. Dimethyl sulfoxide (DMSO)—a status report. Clinical Medicine. 78:21-31.

John, H. and G. Laudahn, 1967. Clinical experiences with the topical application of DMSO in orthopedic diseases: Evaluation of 4180 cases. Ann. N.Y. Acad. Sci. 141(1): 506-516.

Kamiya, S., Wakao, T. and K. Nishioka, 1966. Studies on improvement of eye drops. III. Bacteriological consideration of DMSO. J. Clin. Phthal. (Jap.) 20:143.

Kappert, A., 1975. Experimental and clinical evaluation of topical dimethyl sulfoxide in venous disorders of the extremities. Ann.

N.Y. Acad. Sci. 243:403-407.

Kharasch, N. and B. S. Thyagarajan, 1966. The chemistry of dimethyl sulfoxide for the period 1961-1965. Quarterly reports of sulfur chemestry. 1(1):1-91.

Kim, S. E. and W. S. Moos, 1967. Radiation protection by topical DMSO application. Health Phys. 13:601-606.

Kleberger, K. E., 1967. An opthalmological evaluation of DMSO. Ann. N.Y. Acad. Sci. 141(1):381-385.

Kligman, A. M., 1965. Topical pharmacology and toxicology of dimethyl sulfoxide—Part 1. JAMA 193(10):796-804.

Kligman, A. M., 1965. Dimethyl sulfoxide—Part 2. JAMA 193(11):923-928.

Kocsis, J. J., Harkaway, S. and R. Snyder, 1975. Biological effects of the metabolites of dimethyl sulfoxide. Ann. N.Y. Acad. Sci. 243:104-109.

Kolb, K. H., Jänicke, G., Kramer, M., Schulze, P. E. and G. Raspe, 1965. Das verhalten von $^{35}S$ markiertem dimethylsulfoxid in menschlichen und tierischen organismus. Arzneimittel-Forsch. 15:1292-1295.

Kolb, K. H. and G. Jänicke, 1966. Weitere untersuchungen zur pharmakokinetik von radioaktiv markiertem DMSO. In: Dimethylsulfoxyd—DMSO. Internationales Symposium. (Eds. G. Laudahn and K. Gertich), Wein. Saladruck, Berlin. pp. 9-13.

Kolb, K. H., Jaenicke, G., Kramer, M. and P. E. Schulze, 1967. Absorption, distribution and elimination of labeled dimethyl sulfoxide in man and animals. Ann. N.Y. Acad. Sci. 141(1):85-95.

Krzywicki, J. and H. Rewerska, 1966. Preliminary evaluation of the usefulness of DMSO (dimethyl sulfoxide) in infectious conditions of the periodontium. Czas. Stomat. XIX, 3:303-304.

Kunze, M., 1975. Production of interferon in the white mouse by dimethyl sulfoxide. Ann. N.Y. Acad. Sci. 243:308-310.

LaHann, T. R. and A. Horita, 1975. Effects of dimethyl sulfoxide (DMSO) on prostaglandin synthetase. Proc. West. Pharmacol. Soc. 18:81-82.

Laudahn, G. and K. Gertich, 1966. Dimethylsulfoxyd—DMSO. Internationales Symposium, Wein. Saladruck, Berlin, 1966. 219 p.

Leake, C. D., 1975. Opening remarks. Ann. N.Y. Acad. Sci. 243:5-6.

Lessler, M. A., Jensen, J. H. and R. B. Berggren, 1973. Effect of cryostorage on oxygen uptake and autograft viability of rat skin. Cryobiology. 10:185-189.

Litvan, G. G., 1972. Mechanism of cryoinjury in biological systems. Cryobiology. 9:182.

Litvinchuk, M. D. and V. V. Nevelichuk, 1972. Towards a pharmacology of dimethylsulfoxidide. Fasmack. Toxa. 35(6):727-731.

Lohmann, W. and A. J. Moss, 1966. Radioprotective effect of DMSO on lactate dehydrogenase. Naturwissenschaften. 53(24):702.

Lovelock, J. E. and M. W. H. Bishop, 1959. Prevention of freezing damage to living cells by dimethyl sulphoxide. Nature, 183:1394-1395.

MacGregor, W. S., 1967. The chemical and physical properties of DMSO. Ann. N.Y. Acad. Sci. 141(1):3-12.

Maddock, C. L., Green, M. N. and B. L. Brown, 1966. Topical administration of anti-tumor agents to locally implanted neoplasma. Proc. Am. A. Cancer Res. 7:46.

Mailbach, H. I. and R. J. Feldmann, 1967. The effect of DMSO on percutaneous penetration of hydrocortisone and testosterone in man. Ann. N.Y. Acad. Sci. 141(1):423-427.

Marin, R. E., 1975. Evaluation of dimethyl sulfoxide therapy in chronic respiratory insufficiency of bronchopulmonary origin. Ann. N.Y. Acad. Sci. 243:475-484.

Marks, P. A. and R. A. Rifkind, 1978. Erythroleukemic differentiation. Ann. Rev. Biochem. 47:419-448.

Marks, P. A., Rifkind, R. A., Bank, A., Terada, M., Gambari, R., Fibach, E., Maniatis, G. and R. Reuben, 1979. Expression of globin genes during induced erythroleukemia cell differentiation. In: Cellular and molecular regulation of hemoglobin switching. (Eds. G. Staniatory-annopoulos and A. W. Neinhuis) Grune and Stratton, New York, pp. 437-455.

Mason, M. M., 1971. Toxicology of DMSO in animals. In: Dimethyl sulfoxide, basic concepts of DMSO. Vol. 1 (Eds. S. W. Jacob, E. E. Rosenbaum and D. C. Wood), Marcel Dekker, Inc., New York, pp. 113-131.

Matsumoto, J., 1967. Clinical trials of dimethyl sulfoxide in rheumatoid arthritis patients in Japan. Ann. N.Y. Acad. Sci. 141(1):560-568.

McDermot, H. L., Finkbeiner, A. J. and B. Zanette, 1967. The fate of dimethyl sulfoxide applied to the skin of the rat. Can. J. Physiocol. and Pharmacol. 45:475-478.

McGrady, P., 1973. The persecuted drug: The study of DMSO. Charter Books, New York, 306 p.

Mellville, K. I., Klinger, B. and H. E. Shisten, 1968. Effects of dimethyl sulfoxide (DMSO) on cardiovascular responses to ouabain proscillaridin and digitoxin. Arch. Int. Pharmacodyn. 174:277-293.

Merck Index, 1976. Dimethyl sulfoxide. Merck Index, 9th ed. (Ed. M. Windholz), Merck and Company, Rahway, 433 p.

Meryman, H. T., 1971. Osmotic stress as a mechanism of freezing injury. Cryobiology. 8:489.

Miranda-Tirado, R., 1975. Dimethyl sulfoxide therapy in chronic ckin ulcers. Ann. N.Y. Acad. Sci. 243:408-411.

Misch, D. W. and M. S. Misch, 1975. The effect of dimethyl sulfoxide on a lysonal membrane. Ann. N.Y. Acad. Sci. 243:54-59.

Nachbar, B., 1972. Clinical investigation of the effectiveness of phlebolan spray in the treatment of aseptic superficial thrombophlebitis. Schwelz. Rundschau. Med. (Praxis) 61:1305-1307.

Nash, T., 1966. Chemical constitution and physical properties of compounds able to protect living cells against damage due to freezing and thawing. In: Cryobiology (Ed. H. T. Meryman), Academic, New York, pp. 179-211.

National Academy of Science-National Research Council, 1973. Dimethyl sulfoxide as a therapeutic agent. Report of the *ad hoc* committee on dimethyl sulfoxide. PB-224-574:1-119.

Noel, P. R. B., Barnett, K. C., Davies, R. E., Jolly, D. W., Leahy, J. S., Mawdesley-Thomas, L. E., Shillam, K. W. G., Squires, P. F., Street, A. E., Tucker, W. D. and A. N. Worden, 1975. The toxicity of dimethyl sulfoxide (DMSO) for the dog, pig, and rabbit. Tox. 3:143-169.

Ogden, H. D., 1967. Experiences with DMSO in treatment of headache. Ann. N.Y. Acad. Sci. 141(1):646-648.

Parsons, J. L., Shepard, W. L. and W. M. Fosdick, 1967. DMSO as an adjunct to physical therapy in the chronic frozen shoulder. Ann. N.Y. Acad. Sci. 141(1):569-571.

Paul, M. M., 1967. Interval therapy with disulfoxide. Ann. N.Y. Acad. Sci. 141(1): 586-598.

Penrod, D. S., Bacharach, B. and J. Y. Templeton, 1967. Dimethyl sulfoxide for incisional pain after thoracotomy: Preliminary report. Ann. N.Y. Acad. Sci. 141(1):493-495.

Perlman, F. and H. F. Wolfe, 1966. Dimethylsulfoxide as a penetrant carrier of allergens through intact human skin. J. Allergy 38:299.

Persky, L. and B. H. Stewart, 1967. The use of dimethyl sulfoxide in the treatment of genitourinary disorders. Ann. N.Y. Acad. Sci. 141(1):551-554.

Peterson, C. G. and R. D. Robertson, 1967. A pharmacodynamic study of dimethyl sulfoxide. Ann. N.Y. Acad. Sci. 141(1):273-276.

Porter, D. M. and W. S. Brey, 1967. A neuclear magnetic resonance study of hydrogen bonding in the succinimide-dimethyl sulfoxide system. J. Phys. Chem. 71(12):3779-3783.

Raettig, H., 1966. Moglichkeiten des DMSO in der experimentellen immunologie. In: Dimethylsulfoxyd—DMSO. Internationales Symposium. (Eds. G. Laudahn and K. Gertich), Wein. Saladruck, Berlin. pp. 51-56.

Ramirez, E. and S. Luza, 1967. Dimethyl sulfoxide in the treatment of mental patients. Ann. N.Y. Acad. Sci. 141(1):655-667.

Rammler, D. H., 1971. Use of DMSO in enzyme-catalyzed reactions. In: Dimethyl sulfoxide, basic concepts of DMSO. Vol. 1 (Eds. S. W. Jacob, E. E. Rosenbaum and D. C. Wood), Marcel Dekker, Inc., New York, pp. 189-206.

Rammler, D. H. and A. Zaffaroni, 1967. Biological implications of DMSO based on a review of its chemical properties. Ann. N.Y. Acad. Sci. 141(1):13-23.

Robinson, J. D., 1975. Specific modifications of the $Na^+$, $K^+$—dependent adenosine triphosphatase by dimethyl sulfoxide. Ann. N.Y. Acad. Sci. 243:60-72.

Rosen, H., Blumenthal, A., Panascvich, R. and J. McCallum, 1965. Dimethyl sulfoxide (DMSO) as a solvent in acute toxicity determinations. Proc. Soc. Exper. Biol. and Med., 120:511.

Rosenbaum, E. E. and S. W. Jacob, 1964. Dimethyl sulfoxide (DMSO) in acute musculoskeletal injuries and inflammations. I. Dimethyl sulfoxide in acute subdeltoid bursitis. N. W. Med. 63:167-168.

Rosenbaum, E. E., Herschler, R. J. and S. W. Jacob, 1965. Dimethyl sulfoxide in musculoskeletal disorders. JAMA 192(4):309-313.

Rosenkrantz, H., Hadidian, Z., Seay, H. and M. M. Mason, 1963. Dimethyl sulfoxide: Its steroid solubility and endocrinologic and pharmacologic characteristics. Cancer Chemother. Rep. 31:7-24.

Roubal, W. T. and A. L. Tappel, 1966. Arch. Biochem. Biophys. 113:5.

Rubin, L. F., 1975. Toxicity of dimethyl sulfoxide, alone and in combination. Ann. N.Y. Acad. Sci. 243:98-103.

Rubin, L. F. and P. A. Mattis, 1966. Dimethyl sulfoxide: Lens changes in dogs during oral administration. Science, 153:83-84.

Sams, W. M., 1967. The effects of dimethyl sulfoxide on nerve conduction. Ann. N.Y. Acad. Sci. 141(1):242-247.

Sams, W. M., Carroll, N. V. and P. L. Crantz, 1966. DMSO bei spondylogen neuropathien. In: Dimethylsulfoxyd—DMSO. Internationales Symposium (Eds. G. Laudahn and K. Gertich), Wein. Saladruck, Berlin, pp. 134-139.

Sandborn, E. B., Stephens, H. and M. Bendayan, 1975. The influence of dimethyl sulfoxide on cellular ultrastructure and cytochemestry. Ann. N.Y. Acad. Sci. 243:122-138.

Sanders, M., 1967. Discussion (On the N.Y. Acad. Sci. Conf. on DMSO) Ann. N.Y. Acad. Sci. 141(1):649-652.

Saytzeff, A. M., 1867. Ueber die einwirkung von salpetersaure auf schwefelmethyl und schwefelathyl. Justus Liebigs Ann. Chem. 144:148-156.

Scherbel, A. L., McCormack, L. J. and J. K. Layle, 1967. Further observations on the effect of dimethyl sulfoxide in patients with generalized scleroderma (progressive systemic sclerosis). Ann. N.Y. Acad. Sci. 141(1):613-629.

Scherbel, A. L., McCormack, L. J. and M. J. Poppo, 1965. Alterations of collagen in generalized scleroderma after treatment with dimethylsulfoxide. Cleveland Clinic Quart. 32:47.

Schrek, R., Elrod, L. M. and K. V. Batra, 1967. Cytocidal effect of dimethyl sulfoxide on normal and leukemic lymphocytes. Ann. N.Y. Acad. Sci. 141(1):202-213.

Sergayev, V. P. and R. Z. Zakiev, 1976. Treatment of scleroderma with dimethyl sulfoxide. Vestn. Dermatol. Venerol. (3):70.

Sehtman, L., 1975. Dimethyl sulfoxide therapy in various dermatological disorders. Ann. N.Y. Acad. Sci. 243:395-402.

Seibert, F. B., Farrelly, F. K. and C. C. Shepherd, 1967. DMSO and other combatants against bacteria isolated from leukemia and cancer patients. Ann. N.Y. Acad. Sci. 141(1): 175-201.

Shilkin, K. B., Papadimitriou, J. M. and M. N. Walters, 1966. The effect of dimethyl sulphoxide on hepatic cells of rats. Australian J. Exptl. Biol. Med. Sci. 44:581.

Skog, E. and J. E. Wahlberg, 1967. Effect of dimethyl sulfoxide on skin. Acta dermvenereol. 47:426-434.

Smith, E. R., Hadidian, Z. and M. M. Mason, 1967. The single—and repeated—dose toxicity of dimethyl sulfoxide. Ann. N.Y. Acad. Sci. 141(1):96-109.

Smith, E. R., Hadidian, Z. and M. M. Mason, 1968. The toxicity of single and repeated dermal applications of dimethyl sulfoxide. J. Clin. Pharmacol. pp. 315-321.

Smith, E. R., Mason, M. M., and E. Epstein, 1969. The ocular effects of repeated dermal applications of dimethyl sulfoxide to dogs and monkeys. J. Pharmacol. Exp. Ther. 170(2):364-370.

Sommer, S. and G. Tauberger, 1973. Toxicologic investigations of dimethyl sulfoxide. Arzneimittel-Forsch. 14:1050-1053.

Spiker, B., 1972. Pharmacological studies on dimethyl sulfoxide. Arch. Int. Pharmacodyn. Ther. 200:153-167.

Steinberg, A., 1967. The employment of dimethyl sulfoxide as an antiinflammatory agent and steroid-transporter in diversified clinical disease. Ann. N.Y. Acad. Sci. 141(1):532-550.

Stewart, G. and S. W. Jacob, 1965. Use of dimethyl sulfoxide (DMSO) in the treatment of post-amputation pain. Amer. Surg. 31(7):460-462.

Steward, B. H. and S. W. Shirley, 1976. Further experience with intravesical dimethyl sulfoxide in the treatment of interstitial cystitis. J. Urol. 116(1):36-38.

Stoughton, R. B. and W. Fritsch, 1964. Influence of dimethylsulfoxide (DMSO). Arch. Derm. 90:515-517.

Sweat, F. W. and W. W. Epstein, 1967. Dimethyl sulfoxide oxidations. J. Org. Chem. 32:835-838.

Szmant, H. H., 1971. Chemistry of DMSO. In: Dimethyl sulfoxide, basic concepts of DMSO. Vol. 1 (Eds. S. W. Jacob, E. E. Rosenbaum and D. C. Wood), Marcel Dekker, Inc. N.Y. pp. 1-97.

Szmant, H. H., 1975. Physical properties of dimethyl sulfoxide and its function in biological systems. Ann. N.Y. Acad. Sci. 243:20-23.

Tiru-Chelvam, R., 1974. The effects of dimethyl sulfoxide on snake venom toxicity in vivo and on the efficacy of antivenins. Curr. Ther. Res. 16(9):1033-1038.

de la Torre, J. C., 1970. Relative penetration of ℓ-dopa and 5-HTP through the brain barrier using dimethyl sulfoxide. Experentia 26:1117-1118.

de la Torre, J. C., 1970. Versatile drug may heal CNS injuries. Univ. Chicago Reports. 26(1):1-3.

de la Torre, J. C., Kawanaga, H. M., Rowed, D. W., Johnson, C. M., Goode, D. J., Kajihara, K. and S. Mullan, 1975. Dimethyl sulfoxide in central nervous system trauma. Ann. N.Y. Acad. Sci. 243:362-389.

de la Torre, J. C. and D. W. Rowed, 1974. DMSO: A new respiratory stimulant? J. Clin. Pharamcol. 14:345-353.

Tsuchiya, T., Iriyama, S. and S. Umezawa, 1964. The formation of methyl methanethiolsulfonate, an antibacterial substance, from dimethyl sulfoxide. Bull. Chem. Soc. Japan. 37:286-287.

Venegas, H., 1975. Dimethyl sulfoxide therapy in sterility due to tubal obstruction. Ann. N.Y. Acad. Sci. 243:491-493.

Vogin, E., Carson, S., Cannon, G., Linegar, C. R. and L. F. Rubin, 1970. Chronic toxicity of DMSO in primates. Toxic Appl. Pharmac. 16:606-612.

Walker, T. M., Albrigo, J. L. and J. A. Panuska, 1966. The effect of dimethylsulfoxide on oxygen consumption in cold-exposed rats and hamsters. Cryobiology. 2:265-268.

Warren, J., Sacksteder, R., Jarosz, H., Wassweman, B. and P. E. Andreotti, 1975. Potentiation of antimeoplastic compounds by oral dimethyl sulfoxide in tumor-bearing rats. Ann. N.Y. Acad. Sci. 243:194-208.

Weaver, W. J., Hill, R. V., Weber, F. S. and S. W. Jacob, 1975. The penetration and clearance of dimethyl sulfoxide from the rat eye after topical application. Ann. N.Y. Acad. Sci. 243:151-154.

Weisman, G., Sessa, G. and V. Bevans, 1967. Effect of DMSO on the stabilization of lysosomes by cortisone and chloroquine in vitro. Ann. N.Y. Acad. Sci. 141(1):326-332.

Weyer, E. M., Hutchins, H., Krauss, M. and C. D. Leake, 1967. Biological actions of dimethyl sulfoxide. Ann. N.Y. Acad. Sci. 141(1):1-671.

Widmer, L. K., Glaus, L. and E. Raps, 1972. Local treatment of leg complaints and chronic venous insufficiency. Schwelz. Rundschau Med. (Praxis) 61:1300-1304.

Williams, K. I. H., Whittemore, K. S., Mellin, T. N. and D. S. Layne, 1965. Oxidation of dimethyl sulfoxide to dimethyl sulfone in the rabbit. Science, 149:203-204.

Willson, J. E., Brown, D. E. and E. K. Timmens, 1965. A toxicologic study of dimethyl sulfoxide. Toxic. Appl. Pharmac. 7:104-112.

Wolfred, M. M., 1966. Pharmacological and toxicological aspects of dimethyl sulfoxide. Quart. Rept. Sulfur Chem. 1:83.

Wood, D. C., 1971. Fate and metabolism of DMSO. In: Dimethyl sulfoxide, basic concepts of DMSO. Vol. 1 (Eds. S. W. Jacob, E. E. Rosenbaum and D. C. Wood), Marcel Dekker, Inc., New York, pp. 133-145.

Wood, D. C., Sweet, D., VanDolah, J., Smith, J. C. and I. Contaxis, 1967. A study of DMSO and steroids in rabbit eyes. Ann. N.Y. Acad. Sci. 141(1):346-380.

Wood, D. C., Weber, F. S. and M. A. Palmquist, 1971. Continued studies in the toxicology of dimethyl sulfoxide (DMSO). J. Pharmacol. Exp. Ther. 177(3):520-527.

Wood, D. C. and J. Wood, 1975. Pharmacologic and biochemical consideration of dimethyl sulfoxide. Ann. N.Y. Acad. Sci. 243:7-19.

Young, H. F., Becker, D. P., Jane, J. A. and F. E. Nulsen, 1968. Mechanism of action of dimethyl sulphoxide. Surg. Forum. 19:439-441.

Zuñiga, A. C., 1975. Dimethyl sulfoxide therapy in subjective tinnitus of unknown origin. Ann. N.Y. Acad. Sci. 243:468-474.

Zuñiga, A., Burdach, R. and S. Rubio, 1975. Dimethyl sulfoxide therapy in bronchiolitis. Ann. N.Y. Acad. Sci. 243:460-467.

# Index

## A



## B



## C



## D

## N



## O



## P



## R



## S

## T



## U



## V



## W-X